PUBLIC HEALTH IN THE 21ST CENTURY SERIES

THE MAKING OF A GOOD DOCTOR

PUBLIC HEALTH IN THE 21ST CENTURY SERIES

Family History of Osteoporosis
Afrooz Afghani (Editor)
2009. ISBN: 978-1-60876-190-6

Cross Infections: Types, Causes and Prevention
Jin Dong and Xun Liang (Editors)
2009. ISBN: 978-1-60741-467-4

Health-Related Quality of Life
Erik C. Hoffmann (Editor)
2009. ISBN: 978-1-60741-723-1

Swine Flu and Pig Borne Diseases
Viroj Wiwanitkit
2009. ISBN: 978-1-60876-291-0

Biological Clocks: Effects on Behavior, Health and Outlook
Oktav Salvenmoser and Brigitta Meklau (Editors)
2010. ISBN: 978-1-60741-251-9

Infectious Disease Modelling Research Progress
Jean Michel Tchuenche and C. Chiyaka (Editors)
2010. ISBN: 978-1-60741-347-9

Firefighter Fitness: A Health and Wellness Guide
Ernest L. Schneider
2010. ISBN: 978-1-60741-650-0

The Making of a Good Doctor
B. D. Kirkcaldy, R. J. Shephard and R. G. Siefen
2010. ISBN: 978-1-60876-449-5

PUBLIC HEALTH IN THE 21ST CENTURY SERIES

THE MAKING OF A GOOD DOCTOR

**B. D. KIRKCALDY
R. J. SHEPHARD
AND
R. G. SIEFEN**

Nova Science Publishers, Inc.
New York

Copyright © 2010 by Nova Science Publishers, Inc.

All rights reserved. No part of this book may be reproduced, stored in a retrieval system or transmitted in any form or by any means: electronic, electrostatic, magnetic, tape, mechanical photocopying, recording or otherwise without the written permission of the Publisher.

For permission to use material from this book please contact us:
Telephone 631-231-7269; Fax 631-231-8175
Web Site: http://www.novapublishers.com

NOTICE TO THE READER

The Publisher has taken reasonable care in the preparation of this book, but makes no expressed or implied warranty of any kind and assumes no responsibility for any errors or omissions. No liability is assumed for incidental or consequential damages in connection with or arising out of information contained in this book. The Publisher shall not be liable for any special, consequential, or exemplary damages resulting, in whole or in part, from the readers' use of, or reliance upon, this material. Any parts of this book based on government reports are so indicated and copyright is claimed for those parts to the extent applicable to compilations of such works.

Independent verification should be sought for any data, advice or recommendations contained in this book. In addition, no responsibility is assumed by the publisher for any injury and/or damage to persons or property arising from any methods, products, instructions, ideas or otherwise contained in this publication.

This publication is designed to provide accurate and authoritative information with regard to the subject matter covered herein. It is sold with the clear understanding that the Publisher is not engaged in rendering legal or any other professional services. If legal or any other expert assistance is required, the services of a competent person should be sought. FROM A DECLARATION OF PARTICIPANTS JOINTLY ADOPTED BY A COMMITTEE OF THE AMERICAN BAR ASSOCIATION AND A COMMITTEE OF PUBLISHERS.

LIBRARY OF CONGRESS CATALOGING-IN-PUBLICATION DATA
Kirkcaldy, Bruce D. (Bruce David), 1952-
 The making of a good doctor / authors, Kirkcaldy, B.D., Shephard, R.J., Siefen, R.G.
   p. ; cm.
 Includes bibliographical references and index.
 ISBN 978-1-60876-449-5 (hardcover)
 1. Medicine--Practice. 2. Physicians. 3. Medical anthropology. I. Shephard, Roy J. II. Siefen, R. G. III. Title.
 [DNLM: 1. Physician's Role. 2. Education, Medical. 3. Physician-Patient Relations. 4. Physicians--psychology. 5. Physicians--standards. 6. Quality of Health Care. W 62 K59m 2009]   R728.K545 2009   610--dc22   2009040817

Published by Nova Science Publishers, Inc. ✦ *New York*

Contents

Chapter 1	Introduction	1
Chapter 2	Anthropological Influences and Resultant Lifestyle Issues	3
Chapter 3	Cross-Cultural Comparisons	7
Chapter 4	Treatment of the Psyche Versus Organic Disease	13
Chapter 5	Patient Assessments of the Quality of Practice	17
Chapter 6	Physician Assessments of Good Practice	23
Chapter 7	Motivators, Stressors, Job Satisfaction and Personal Qualities of a Good Physician	25
Chapter 8	Economic Assessments of the Quality of Health Care	33
Chapter 9	Selection and Training of Medical Students	41
Chapter 10	Monitoring and Maintenance of Personal Health	47
Chapter 11	Medical Doctors in the Focus of Attention and of Contradictory Interests in Health Care	59
Chapter 12	Conclusions	61
References		63
Contributors		73
Index		75

My thanks to my youngest daughter, Eliana, who continues to teach me with lively mid-day conversations. And to my eldest daughter Lisenka who persists in pursuing her passion, and my wife Lisa. BDK.

My thanks to my family- Muriel, Sarah and Rachel- for all of their patience in my writing endeavours. RJS.

Gratitude to my wife Friederike and my son Janko, who always encourage me to do research, teach and work in the best interest of patients and their families. RGS.

Chapter 1

INTRODUCTION

"The good physician treats the disease. The great physician treats the patient who has the disease" (William Osler)

"It seems to me that medicine has indulged in a Faustian bargain. A three-thousand year tradition, which bonded doctor and patient in a special affinity of trust, is being traded for a new type of relationship. Healing is replaced with treating, care is supplanted by managing, and the art of listening is taken over by technological procedures. Doctors no longer minister to a distinctive person but concern themselves with fragmented, malfunctioning biological parts. The distressed person is frequently absent from the transaction" (Lown, 1999, p. xiv).

What makes a good doctor? Television and film portrayals are often superficial (Easton, 2006), but the question is brought into sharp focus by the British Independent Television series "Doc. Martin" (2008). In this popular programme, a doctor who had hoped to become a surgeon reacts badly to the sight of blood, and so is forced to become a general practitioner in a small and rather backward Cornish fishing village. He proves himself a brilliant diagnostician. His treatments are rapid and effective, and he never submits to the unreasonable whims of his patients. However, he is very shy and has an abrasive manner of speaking, so that he rapidly alienates almost all of his clientele. This highlights a major issue in the assessment of a physician. Is the doctor's primary objective to establish a good rapport with his or her patient, or is it more important to assess objective evidence of success in terms of a reduced burden of clinical disease in the community that the doctor is serving? Is there a major "disconnect" between the modern emphasis on practicing evidence-based medicine and the subjective qualities on which many patients continue to judge their physicians? Should the personal attributes of a medical practitioner be considered at all, other than in the context of the contribution that they make to meeting the goals of modern, evidence-based medicine? For specialities in disciplines such as psychiatry and psychotherapy, the immediate personal relationship between the physician and the patient is clearly central. But here, too, the quality of care, the appropriateness of interventions and the effectiveness of treatment demand appropriate "benchmarking," much as in other medical specialties.

This article suggests some techniques that can be adopted both to evaluate and to enhance the quality of medical care. A good doctor must pay due attention to cultural and anthropological **factors that influence a patient's lifestyle** and any resulting need to adjust personal lifestyle in the interests of health. Account must be taken of cross-cultural differences **in the patient's expect**ations, accepted patterns of treatment and health outcomes. Often, a family physician must be prepared to address psychological problems rather than the presence of a clear-cut organic disease of the type anticipated by those formulating evidence-based treatment recommendations. The quality of an individual medical practice and levels of health achieved can be rated by both the patients who are treated and peers from the health professions, although the views of both groups must be accepted with caution. Considering the usual motivators, stressors and personal qualities of a successful physician can enhance the quality of any given practice. Finally, on a provincial or a national scale, health outcomes can be weighed against medical expenditures per unit of population. All of these various factors need careful consideration by policy makers in the contexts of physician selection, techniques of medical education and the design of management systems to optimize practice and enhance the skills of individual practitioners. Nevertheless, many of the proposed criteria are complex, changeable and difficult to quantify (Baker, 2006; Wakeford, 2006).

Chapter 2

ANTHROPOLOGICAL INFLUENCES AND RESULTANT LIFESTYLE ISSUES

Humans have undergone a progressive evolutionary adaptation to their immediate environment over many millennia. Illnesses thus arise because the current generation of Homo sapiens no longer maintains the life-style to which it became so well adapted over the centuries. A good physician recognizes the problems inherent in our current urban lifestyle and seeks to maximize the individual's health potential by focussing on preventive medicine and the development of health habits such as exercise and diet that are more appropriate to our constitutional background.

ANTHROPOLOGICAL FACTORS

Earlier generations of humans lived on regionally available natural food products, and of necessity engaged in much vigorous physical activity, either in hunting and gathering or in the cultivation of crops (Shephard & Rode, 1996). But the advent of imported, genetically manipulated and synthetic food products has vastly altered human diets and mechanization and computerization have greatly reduced the need for physical activity either at work or in the home. The current generation thus attempts to live in a world for which it is poorly adapted, with the resultant emergence of many "lifestyle diseases."

Some aspects of an optimal lifestyle are universal. However, it is also helpful to know the specific genetic and culturally-mediated antecedents of a particular patient or group of patients, as some aspects of evolutionary adaptation differ from one habitat to another. For instance, the coastal Inuit have adapted to a diet rich in omega fatty acids, but lacking in lactose (Rode, Shephard, Vloschinsky & Kuksis, 1995); many people in these communities thus have difficulty in metabolizing milk products.

Unfortunately, medical curriculae rarely address either anthropological aspects of health or the issues of lifestyle modification associated with 21st century life. Moreover, doctors too often, lack both the knowledge and the skills to prevent or correct an inappropriate lifestyle. Instead, they opt to treat the symptoms or signs of disease that they have learned in medical school. For example, they may elect to treat obesity by appetite suppressing drugs, and hypertension by hypotensive agents, often with serious side-effects, rather than recommending an increase in physical activity and a reduced food intake (which would be at least as effective a remedy, and would have benefits in other areas of the patient's health). The lifestyle issues underlying common diseases are too frequently completely ignored. Probable reasons for this bias include the doctor's limited knowledge of techniques for enhancing healthy behaviour, and the speed of prescribing a simple chemical remedy in an over-busy clinic. However, a good physician will encourage patients where possible to adopt those features of lifestyle to which humankind has adapted over centuries of evolution.

PREVENTIVE MEDICINE AND PERSONAL LIFESTYLE

The need for a greater focus on preventive medicine has been documented repeatedly. The issue is well illustrated by a longitudinal study of almost 80,000 middle-aged women conducted in the U.S. (Van Dam, Spiegelman, Franco & Hu, 2008). At their initial examination, in 1980, none of the women showed any evidence of cancer or cardiovascular disease. However, over the next 24 years, 28% of deaths were estimated as due to smoking habits alone and 55% were due to some combination of smoking, overweight, inadequate physical activity, and poor diet, all factors that a good physician should have corrected. A demonstrated ability to focus on the prevention and correction of major risk factors is an important indicator of a good physician and it can make a major contribution to population health.

"In contrast to acute and infectious diseases, chronic diseases do not arise suddenly... (they) develop gradually... The natural life history... is one of evolution through stages of susceptibility, early illness and finally advanced or disabling disease. Progress through these three stages may be illustrated with coronary heart disease. At the stage of susceptibility, the individual is healthy, but is exposed to certain health risks.... such as a sedentary life... or cigarette smoking. If these health risks lead to the development of arteriosclerostic plaques.... the individual is at the stage of... preclinical disease in which few, if any, symptoms are present. As the disease advances, it becomes symptomatic..... Angina pectoris and heart attacks are advanced manifestations of coronary heart disease. This natural life history... is not inevitable...." (p.213, Tetrick, Quick and Quick, 2005).

In attempting to modify the lifestyle of a patient, the physician has some advantage over other health care professionals because traditionally, the patient respects his or her authority and the advice that may be offered. However, effectiveness in this area of medical practice also requires an understanding of psychological concepts such as locus of control and behavioural change theory, topics that are rarely taught in medical school. Furnham (1988) asserted that persons with an internal locus of control would exhibit superior adaptive tactics, showing greater responsibility for their health and being careful to avoid potentially dangerous and accident-prone behaviour. They would also try harder to protect themselves from physical illness, and would be more likely to seek comprehensive health care information. Furthermore, they would have a greater awareness of changes in their physiological state and would exert greater self-control over body functions, preferring medical treatments that did not restrict their personal control. Building on previous work by Lau (1982), Kirkcaldy, Shephard and Furnham (2002, p. 1362) suggested that an "Internal locus of control is intimately associated with general health, so that one would expect those with such a locus to be more sensitive to health messages, more keen to enhance their physical health (positive attitudes towards physical exercise and physical activity; increased participation in physical and recreational pursuits, more likely to be non-smokers) and more likely to show psychological well-being".

Chapter 3

CROSS-CULTURAL COMPARISONS

"Anthropologists have demonstrated that different cultures have "prescribed" ways of presenting their illness to others; the language and models they use to describe illness; how to attribute the causes of illness; and the selection, training and monitoring of recognised healers. The medical treatment given in one culture (e.g. placebos) may therefore have quite different effects in a second culture". (p. 123) Furnham (1988).

Cultural factors certainly have a major influence on the perceived health of a patient, health beliefs, expectations concerning the nature of medical treatment, both necessary and unnecessary, and concepts of what it is appropriate for a physician to disclose in terms of diagnosis and prognosis. Various surveys have explored these issues on a national and/or a regional basis, although the relative rankings of countries must be viewed with some caution, since the questions were usually posed in the corresponding national language, and this may have led to some differences of interpretation between respondent groups. Certainly, it is hard to discern any clear patterns or underlying reasons for the apparent differences in response.

PERCEIVED HEALTH

Almost 90 percent of Irish reported enjoying superior health, followed closely by people from Denmark (82%), Netherlands (82%), Belgium (81%), Luxemburg (80%) and Sweden (80%). In contrast, much smaller proportions of those living in Lithuania, Latvia, Estonia and Hungary reported "good or very good" health (European Commission, 2007).

Subjective perceptions of "general health" were highest in Ireland, followed by Greece, Netherlands, Austria, Denmark and Spain, and values were lowest in Portugal, Germany, Finland and Italy (EU, 2007). "Overall health" (a composite index, based on scores for perceived health, chronic morbidity, visual and/or auditory impairment, restrictions of activity through ill-health or impairments of mobility) received low ratings in the UK and Portugal. Netherlands and Austria had the best overall health, followed by Italy, Spain and Greece. Subsequent surveys showed that mental health problems were reported most frequently among the Portuguese and Italians, and least commonly among Finns and Swedes.

REASONS FOR SEEKING TREATMENT

Eurobarometer (2007) asked respondents "For what reasons are you undergoing a long-term medical treatment?" The most commonly stated reason was hypertension (36%), followed by long standing musculo-skeletal problems (rheumatism, arthritis), other conditions (24%), diabetes (15%), chronic anxiety or depression (10%), asthma (9%), osteoporosis (8%), allergies (6%), migraine and frequent headaches (5%), cancer (4%), chronic bronchitis, emphysema (4%), stroke or cerebral haemorrhage (4%) and peptic ulcer (3%). Certain ailments were more common among women, including long-term musculo-skeletal problems (26% vs. 18%), migraine/frequent headaches (22% vs. 11%), chronic anxiety and depression (12% vs. 6%) and osteoporosis (8% vs. 2%).

There were regional differences in the reported reasons for seeking treatment. Hypertension was more frequently cited by those living in East-Central European countries and the Mediterranean. In Romania, Bulgaria, Greece and Slovakia it accounted for a half of individuals undergoing long term treatment, whereas in the Benelux countries it accounted for only a quarter of long-term medical treatment. Over a quarter of Bulgarians reported high blood pressure, closely followed by Lithuanians, Hungarians and Slovakians (25-28%). Allergies were common among Swedes (34%); in contrast, Mediterranean countries – with the exception of Malta - showed a below average proportion of allergies. The likelihood of chronic anxiety or depression was twice the EU average in French respondents; rates were also high in Estonians, but low in Austrians and Slovakians (3%).

REGIONAL DIFFERENCES IN PRESCRIBED MEDICATIONS

Regional differences in the prescription of medications (OECD, 2008) can be illustrated by the sales of medications commonly used in treating mental disorders (Kirkcaldy, 2009). In the figures that follow, the defined daily dosage per 1000 inhabitants was used thus "controlling" for national differences in population size. Analgesics were used more widely in Denmark, Sweden, Norway, Iceland and the United Kingdom and less frequently in the Netherlands, Portugal, Belgium and Germany. Anti-depressant drugs were used most commonly in Iceland, Australia, Sweden and Denmark, and less often in the Slovak Republic, Hungary, Czech Republic and Germany. (Figure 2). Finally, anxiolytics were most likely to be prescribed in Portugal, France, Hungary and Luxemburg, and least likely to be used in Belgium, Germany, Austria and Sweden (Figure 1). National differences in the prescription of these various psycho-pharmaceutical products raise the question of whether there are indeed real differences in the need for such treatment, and whether the prescription is in some instances inappropriate.

GENDER DIFFERENCES

There are important gender differences with respect to the attitudes of both physicians and patients. Buddeberg-Fischer, Stamm, Buddeberg, & Klaghofer (2008) noted that in Switzerland, female physicians had a better appreciation of the need to reconcile the requirements of family and professional working life than did their male peers. The lesser income and status commonly associated with family medicine led to recruitment of fewer career-oriented applicants. In contrast, practitioners in prestigious specialities showed a high level of competitiveness, and such employment was more appealing to male doctors.

Furnham & Kirkcaldy (1997) noted that complementary forms of medical treatment were sought more by female than by male patients, and that overall "women adopt a more critical stance towards doctors because of multiple, more complex, behaviourally oriented ailments and their recognition that general practitioners who adopt a predominantly physical model of illness are unable to cope adequately with women's complaints" (Furnham & Kirkcaldy, 1997, p. 66).

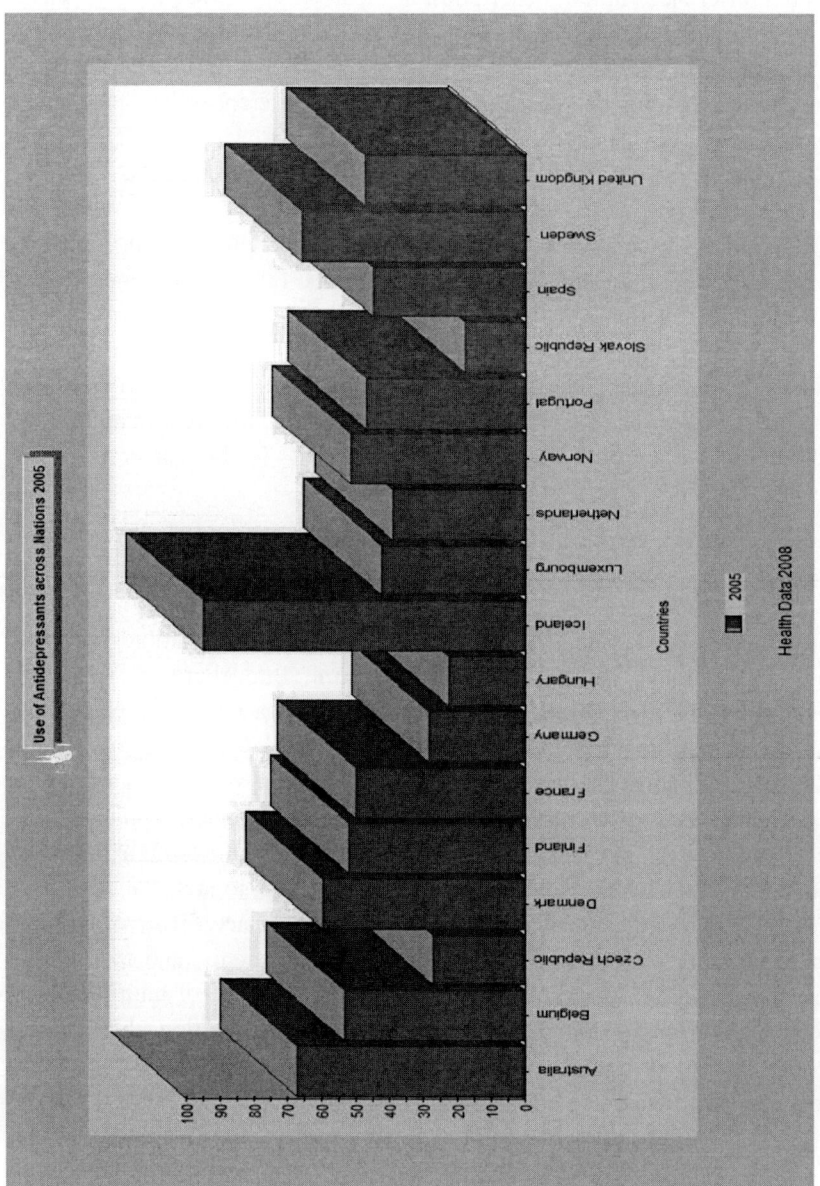

Figure 1. Use of Antidepressants (ddd – defined daily dosage per 1000 inhabitants per day) across some OECD Countries in 2005
Source: "OECD Health Data 2008, December 08, OECD, Paris"

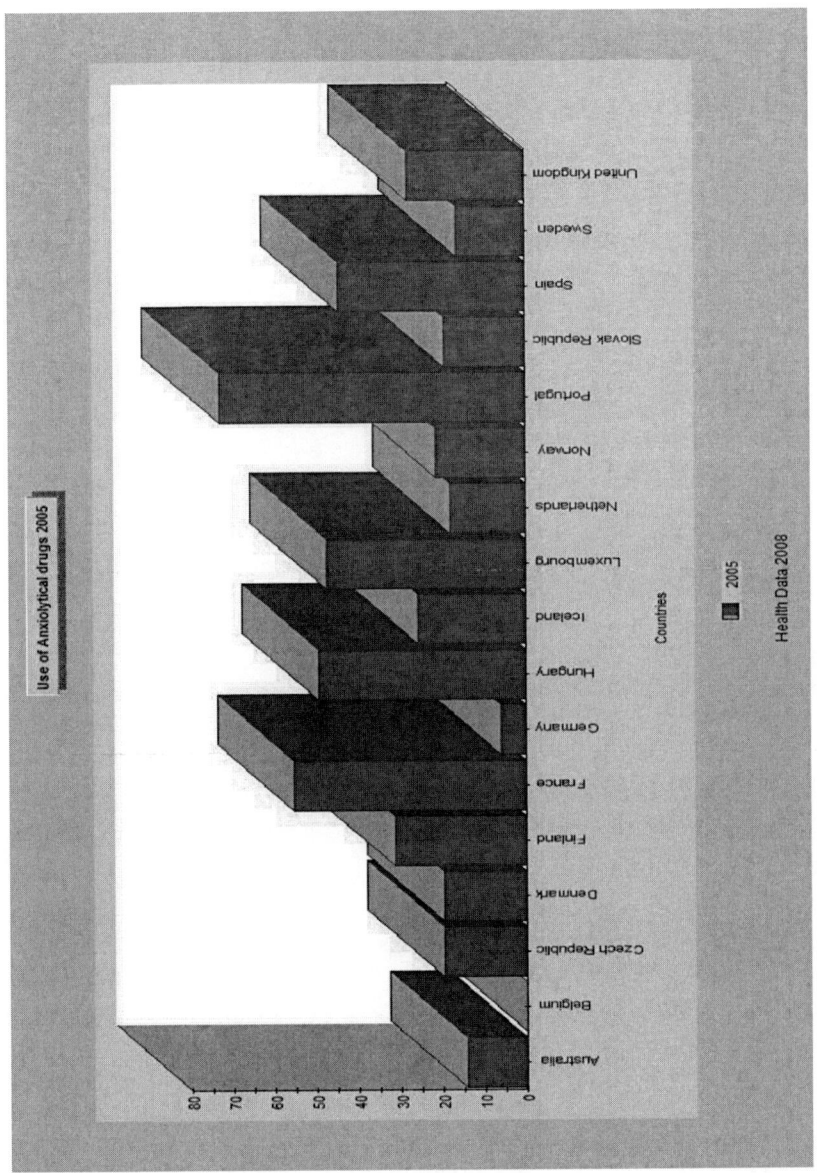

Figure 2. Use of Anxiolytical drugs (ddd – defined daily dosage per 1000 inhabitants per day) across some OECD Countries in 2005. source: "OECD Health Data 2008, December 08, OECD, Paris"

ISSUES IN TRADITIONAL SOCIETIES

Physicians must finally take due account of specific issues that arise in certain traditional societies. In some cultures, medical treatment is viewed as a form of "performance" (Sokol, 2008). One interesting example is the Navajo belief that language and thought impinge on future events. In consequence, Navajo patients perceive that open discussion of a bad prognosis damages their chances of recovery, in essence creating a self-fulfilling prophecy (Sokol, 2004).

Chapter 4

TREATMENT OF THE PSYCHE VERSUS ORGANIC DISEASE

Classical medical training has focussed on the diagnosis and treatment of organic disease rather than the psychological problems of a patient. But particularly in general practice, an ability to operate in the domain of psychology is an important asset. A good family physician should be astute in identifying psychological dysfunction, especially chronic depression and/or substance abuse – which together account for up to 90 percent of suicides.

"In the land of the sick, emotions reign supreme.... our mental well-being is based in part on the illusion of invulnerability. Sickness – especially a severe illness – bursts that illusion, attacking the premise that our private world is safe and secure...The problem is when medical personnel ignore how patients are reacting *emotionally*..., **people's emotional** states can play a sometimes significant role in their vulnerability to disease and in the course of their recovery" (p.164-165, Goleman 1996). "**For the patient, any encounter with a nurse** or physician can be a chance for reassuring information, comfort, and solace – or, if handled unfortunately, an invitation to despair... To be sure, there are compassionate nurses and physicians who take the time to reassure and inform as well as administer medically. But the trend is toward a professional universe in which institutional imperatives can leave medical staff oblivious to the vulnerabilities of patients... With the hard realities of a medical system increasingly timed by accountants, things seem to be getting worse" (p. 165, Goleman, 1996).

Doctors must frequently determine whether an ailment has a "somatic" or a psychological basis, or both. Individuals with somatic illness often display increased anxiety and depression, and there is commonly a bi-directional relationship between negative affect and a physical ailment (Leue, van OS,

Neeleman, de Graf, Vollebergh & Stockbrügger, 2005). Kirkcaldy and co-workers noted consistently positive correlations between scales purporting to measure physical and psychological health (0.53 for managerial staff, 0.48 for paramedical professions, and 0.60 for medical directors) (Kirkcaldy & Cooper, 1992; Kirkcaldy & Shephard, 2001 and Kirkcaldy & Siefen, 2002).

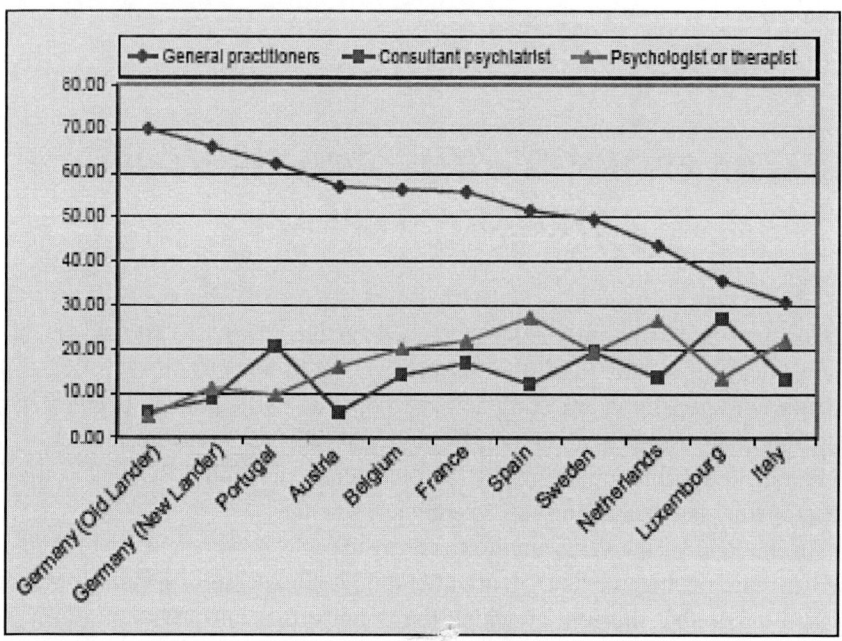

Source: Eurobarometer, October 2002

Figure 3. The source of psychological advice for Europeans in 2002. Types of health providers consulted for mental health problems during the previous year (Source EU, 2007)

An abundant literature testifies to the need for the general practitioner to demonstrate expertise in elementary psychology. In any given year, about a quarter of the US adult population suffers from some form of mental disturbance. Overall, a similar proportion of Europeans (27%) develop mental disorders, with 10-16% of the population seeking treatment for a psychological problem in any given year. The percentage of such consultations is higher in France, the Netherlands and Belgium, and lower in Italy, Spain and Austria (Figure 3).

Women are more likely to seek psychological help than men – possibly, they are more susceptible to psychological disorders, or possibly men are less willing to disclose emotional vulnerability. However, some countries did not show gender differences in GP consultations for mental health problems e.g. Italy, Netherlands and Spain. Overall, most European patients consult their general practitioner if they perceive that they have a mental health problem. The likelihood of a GP facing such a consultation was greatest in Great Britain, France and N. Ireland, and least in Italy, Greece and Finland. Psychiatric specialists were more likely to be consulted in Portugal and Luxemburg, whereas in Spain, the Netherlands Italy, France and Belgium, patients were likely to consult a psychologist/therapist (Figure 3 & 4).

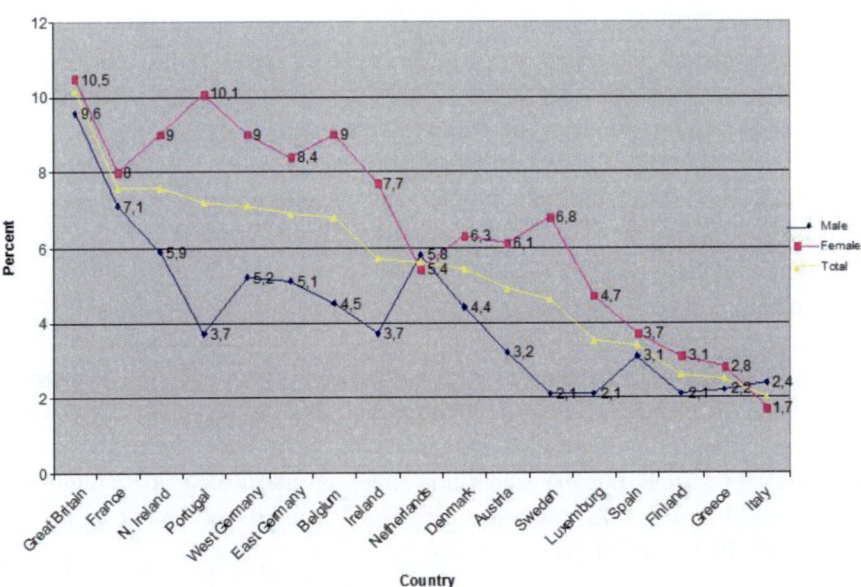

Figure 4. Source - The percentage of Europeans seeking treatment for medical problems in 2002 (Data drawn from Source: Eurobarometer 2002)

Livingston (2006) illustrates the type of problem the family doctor may face. "A patient who appeared in my office recently was a veteran of several psychiatrists and a consumer of considerable medication. He listed his problems as follows: "anxiety, depression, attention deficit disorder, insomnia, sleep apnoea, and narcolepsy". **He was, of course, taking antidepressants** and anti-anxiety agents. In addition, he was on methamphetamine for an acute depressive disorder and hypnotic medicine to help him sleep. He had surgery on his soft palate to help with snoring and was hooked up to a positive pressure machine every night to insure that he didn't stop breathing in his sleep. He wasn't much interested in psychotherapy. ...This is not to deny that medication is frequently invaluable to help people deal with mental illness:.... Medicines can also help temporarily with problems in living: situational anxiety, grief, posttraumatic stress. But when *the only thing* psychiatrists do for people is medicate them for their intrapsychic discomforts, we have sacrificed something essential in our professional identities. We also convey the message... that the passive acceptance of such "treatment" is the preferred method of dealing with emotional problems. I prefer to challenge people to relinquish passivity, stop waiting for answers outside themselves, mobilise their courage and determination, and try and discover what changes will bring them closer to others and to the people they want to be" (p.39-41, Livingston, 2006).

Specific mental and behavioral disorders currently account for some 9% of all medical expenditures (OECD; 2008). One of the most distressing manifestations of mental ill-health is suicide. The WHO (2009) noted an annual total of 1 million suicides and 10-20 million attempted suicides world-wide. The incidence varies substantially from one country to another, rates being highest in Korea, Japan and Hungary and lowest in Greece, Italy, Spain, the UK and Mexico.

"When psychological problems dominate an illness, as is commonly the case, the general physician often diagnoses psychoneurosis, a wastebasket term to which are consigned a host of conditions lacking scientific explanations. The patient is seriously short-changed by this dismissal of the psychological aspects of illness, and ignoring the emotional dimension lessens a doctor's capacity to ameliorate a chronic disease. Drugs may improve some of the presenting symptoms for a time, but the underlying illness is not healed. Inattention to the psychological domain fractures medicine at its heart by divorcing curing from healing" (p. 30, Lown, 1999).

Chapter 5

PATIENT ASSESSMENTS OF THE QUALITY OF PRACTICE

"In the case of illness, one's confinement, one's hopes and one's fears, what one hears or believes, one's physician, *his* behaviour, are all coalesced in a single picture or drama" (O. Sacks, 197?, "Awakenings").

"How can lay theories of illness be of practical value in healthcare? Take the example of the medical practitioner-client relationship: it has been shown that medical staff can establish a better relationship with a patient through knowledge of subjective theories. Patients feel more like they are being taken seriously; the gulf between the physician and the patient is narrowed, and an entry to therapy is facilitated. If no agreement between the subjective theories of the physician and the patient is achieved, this can have a negative effect on the therapeutic relationship. This is often a primary cause of non-compliance with therapy on the part of the patient " as has been shown by Amann and Wipplinger (1998) and Becker (1985). (Kirkcaldy et al, 2007, p. 365)

"Social and medical psychologists as well as medical sociologists, have developed a model of mainly Western lay-people's health beliefs. It has been suggested that these health beliefs are better predictors of a person's health behaviour than personality or individual difference variables favoured by psychologists or demographic variables favoured by sociologists, These health beliefs may be better called health understanding, as they concern knowledge, attitudes, values and beliefs (Pendleton, 1983)" p. 111 (Furnham, 1988).

King (1983) proposed a model of health and illness that emphasised subjective perceptions rather than objective medical detail. The main components of this model included *health motivation* (a person's interest and concern about health issues), *perceived susceptibility* (liability to illness and acceptance of others' diagnoses), *perceived severity* (perceived likelihood of the ailment being serious and the social and somatic consequences of being ill and/or left untreated), *benefits and costs* (subjective estimates of the benefits of taking the prescribed medical treatment – particularly the relief of symptoms - compared with the eventual costs – economic, physical and psychological discomfort) and *cues to action* (factors that initiate action/concern for health behaviour such as the illness of a family member, a magazine or journal article, a reminder from a GP, or the detection of a symptom)

"**People have complex beliefs** about health and illness shaped by their personal and social circumstances, their medical history and encounters with professionals. Demographic and psychological factors also play a part in shaping, maintaining and changing health beliefs. There is rich, multidisciplinary literature on the nature and function of health beliefs and how they operate. These beliefs play a part in many health-care decisions and would appear to be important in the **decision to consult and receive treatment (complementary) practitioners**" (Vincent & Furnham, 1997, p. 116).

Lay theories of illness can help to improve many aspects of medical care. Take, for example, the physician–patient relationship. Physicians develop more favourable relationships with patients as they gain a knowledge of subjective theories. Patients feel taken more seriously and the gulf with the doctor is lessened, facilitating entry into and compliance with treatment. Conversely, an absence of consensus between the subjective theories of the physician and the patient may have an adverse effect on treatment. Kirkcaldy et al (2006) underlined the need to understand health attitudes in treating recent immigrants effectively.

"**While the achievements of orthodox** medicine are undoubtedly impressive, many commentators have pointed out the adverse consequences of an increasingly technological approach to medicine and suggested that this might underlie the popularity of more traditional, less technologically based therapies... In most Westernised countries the orthodox medical system is well established, regulated and controlled, but also subject to criticism. Common criticisms are that orthodox medicine has become too technical and has tended to reduce patient autonomy, making them dependent on drugs or surgery. Pfifferling (1980) considers that modern medicine has become too physician-centred in that the doctor, and not the patient, **defines the nature and boundary of the patient's problem: diagnostic and intellectual skills are valued above communication skills; settings for health care, such as doctors' offices, are often located for the benefit of doctors, far from their patients' homes.** " (p. 30, Vincent & Furnham, 1997)

Informal criticisms of medical practice commonly originate with the patient, rather than physicians or the administrators of a health-care system, and indeed the patient carries an ever-greater responsibility for the type and quality of care that he or she receives. "Responsibility for medical care has landed on the shoulders of patients with a resounding thud. I don't mean choice of doctors .. (but) choice about what the doctors *do*. The tenor of medical practice has shifted from one in which the all-knowing, paternalistic doctor tells the patient what must be done – or just does it – to one in which the doctor arrays possibilities before the patient...", (Schwartz, 2005, p.30) Giving patients more responsibility has improved the quality of medical health care, but "patients see choice as both a blessing and a burden. And the burden falls primarily on women, who are typically the guardians not only of their health but that of their husbands and children" (p.30), ... navigation towards medical visits and subsequent diagnoses and treatment will reflect the needs and expectations of patients...., leading to a "diffusion of responsibility" (Schwartz, 2005). One problem if the patient assumes greater personal responsibility is that anxiety about neglecting minor symptoms may lead to over-diagnosis and an over-consumption of medical care. The doctor may then feel obliged to arrange non-essential diagnostic procedures and unnecessary diagnostic referrals, leading to a cost-ineffective escalation of services.

Attitudes and assessments depend greatly on the health beliefs of the individual concerned. In principle, a patient is well-placed to judge the quality of care that he or she receives, and there have been occasional attempts to determine the merit pay of physicians on the basis of reported patient satisfaction (Kmietowicz, 2006). Dominant issues for many patients are confidence and trust in their physician (Robertson, Dixon & LeGrand, 2008). Another important issue for many patients is the ability always to see the same doctor (Potiriadis, Chondros, Gilchrist et al, 2008). Other factors positively related to patient satisfaction include: "practitioners' contact with the patient, empathy, expression of positive affect, the amount and type of information given, and the degree to which patients perceived their expectations to be met. Patients' perception of ... overall competence is naturally a powerful factor... To some extent, these many factors can be reduced to two: warmth and information." (p. 124, Vincent and Furnham, 1997).

In some countries, patient satisfaction is influenced by their ability to see the practitioner of their choice. Belgian, German and Swiss GPs function in an "open market" system, where patients can select their practitioners freely, but in other jurisdictions it is quite difficult to choose or to change physicians. The time allocated to an individual consultation is another question affecting patient satisfaction, and likely the quality of the care that is offered. The average duration of primary care visits differs substantially from one country to another (Deveugele, Derese, van den Brick-Muinen, Benzing, & De Maeseneer, 2002). Figures range from Germany (7.6 min) and the U.K. (9.4 min) to Belgium (15.0 min) and Switzerland (15.6 min). Age and sex of the doctor do not seem to influence session duration, but consultations are generally longer for female patients, especially in urban areas, and where psychosocial problems are involved. A culture of brief consultations is sometimes blamed on the high demand of medical services. German and Spanish physicians currently see in excess of 200 patients per week, and in such a situation even a 15-minute allocation per patient would necessitate a ten-hour working day.

The Health Consumer Powerhouse report (Björnberg & Uhlir, 2008) adopted a novel ranking of health systems in 31 European nations. Thirty four health performance indicators included: patient rights and information (e.g. access to personal records); e-health (e.g. the penetration of electronic records); waiting times for diagnosis and treatment (e.g. direct access to specialist); specific clinical outcomes (e.g. fatality rate for myocardial infarction, infant mortality rate), the range and reach of services (e.g. affordability of dental care, infant vaccination); access to pharmaceuticals. The highest ratings were for the Netherlands, followed by Denmark and Austria. In fourth position was Luxemburg, then Sweden (excellent technical healthcare, but long waiting times) and Germany. Both Germany and Luxemburg offered excellent accessibility of services. France had occupied first position in 2006, but dropped to 10th position because of weaknesses in developing e-Health solutions. The lowest scores were reported for Latvia, FYR Macedonia, Croatia, Bulgaria and Romania.

Despite some inter-survey inconsistencies, questionnaire responses suggest considerable international differences and a rather low overall patient satisfaction with current health care systems. The 2003 World Health Survey reported the greatest level of satisfaction in Austria (70.4% of patients very satisfied), Belgium (50.3%), Denmark (54.4%), France (37.6%) and the UK (35.4%), and the least satisfaction in Slovakia (1.3%), Estonia (2.3%), Latvia (3.9%), Italy (7.2%) and Hungary (8.0%). Mossialos (1996) found somewhat differing results, with the highest levels of patient dissatisfaction (fairly or very dissatisfied) for Italy (59.4%) Portugal (59.3%), Greece (53.9%), UK (42.9%), and Ireland (29.1%); in this survey, satisfaction levels were highest in Finland (86.4%), the Netherlands (72.8%), Luxemburg (70.1%), Sweden (67.3%) and Germany (66.0%). A third survey of EU nations (OECD Health Data, 2008) reported the least satisfaction with the national health system (% of people who think it is "running well") in Portugal (1.8), Greece (2.9), Ireland (3.7), Italy (6.) and the Netherlands (6.5). The highest satisfaction scores were seen in Austria (31.8), Finland (24.0), Belgium (23.8), France (22.0) and Luxemburg (21.7).

Cleary, Edgman-Levitan, Roberts, Moloney, McMullen, Walker, & Delbanco (1991) focussed specifically on the complaints of patients when admitted to hospital. Problems of communication were common in this environment (45% of patients were "not being told about daily routine;" 21% reported that doctors and nurses did not explain how much pain or discomfort could be anticipated before administering a test; 20% stated that hospital staff did not go out of their way to meet the patient's needs). There were also many reports suggesting a lack of emotional support and sensitivity among hospital staff; doctors talked about patients as if they were not there (9.3%), it was difficult to find a staff member who showed concern for them (8.1%), and there was a lack of a trusting relationship with anyone other than the doctor in immediate charge of the patient (38.7%). Nursing care was often poor (28% of patients felt the nurses were overworked and too busy to take care of them; 24% had not been given a clear explanation of the side-effects of their medication), and there was little preparation for discharge (34% had received no instruction about diet; 26% had not been informed of danger signals to watch for, and 24% were not told when they could resume normal activities). In all, 22% of patients had less than five minutes of discussion with the doctor before discharge, and 90% had not been told about their medication and test results in a comprehensible manner. Such problems were particularly prevalent among those who were poor or in inferior health.

Whether in general practice or in hospital, the physician's communication skills are likely to influence ratings of satisfaction with treatment. Simply getting doctors to seek their patient's opinions, allowing patients to disclose their personal stories, and encouraging them to participate actively in their treatment could do much to enhance the quality of health care (Clever, Jin, Levinson & Meltzer, 2008). In this context, the time spent talking to patients emerges as a central parameter. Lown (1999) comments that a patient may turn to medicine to repair "what are essentially tears in the social fabric wrought by violence, economic oppression, class ostracism, racism, sexism, and a host of other factors. In a consumer culture.... medicalization is the response to mounting social frustrations. Dissatisfactions with one's job or marriage or children, or with one's lot in life, are not uncommonly somaticised. Most doctors do not have the time, patience, training, or incentives to become involved in these societal quagmires, and their inattention leads patients to shop around for a quick fix" (p. 317, Lown, 1999).

Patient ratings offer important insights into how a medical system may be improved, but nevertheless must be accepted with considerable caution. Opinions are readily swayed by the externals of a practice - the architecture and decor of the office (Kemsley, 2008), the "bedside manner" of the physician, and the number of laboratory tests and referrals made, rather than the true healing ability of a practitioner. Too often, clinical excellence becomes defined as the ability to treat a patient's illness as he or she defines it. However, there is much more to true clinical skill than either satisfying the whims and desires of the patient in an efficient manner (Ashcroft, 2002) or providing an aura of magic (Gorin Rosenbaum, 2002). Communication skills and the ability to exert a placebo effect are clearly desirable attributes, but they should not be the sole measures of good practice; indeed, verbal skills can sometimes mask frank incompetence (Cumming, 2002).

Chapter 6

PHYSICIAN ASSESSMENTS OF GOOD PRACTICE

Health professionals have often debated among themselves what makes a good doctor (see, for example, General Medical Council, 2001; Royal College of General Practitioners, 2002; Herzig et al. (2006) and the extensive correspondence elicited by the article of Hurwitz and Vass, 2002). Two questions posted on the BMJ website (bmj.com): "what makes a good doctor?" and "how can we make one?" brought responses from over 100 people in 24 countries. The resultant listing of desirable characteristics emphasized subjective inter-personal characteristics such as compassion, understanding, honesty, humanity, competence, commitment, empathy, respect, creativity and a sense of justice (Hurwitz & Vass, 2002). Surprisingly little attention was directed to knowledge of evidence-based medicine or to objectively assessed measures of health, quality of life and treatment outcomes.

In "The Lost Art of Healing", the cardiologist Lown (1999) maintains that a "good doctor" is well-trained in the medical sciences and pursues the latest advances in research; provides a chemistry of compatibility (becomes an "intimate friend" for the patient); shakes the patient's hand on meeting (offering a "gesture of sympathy"); is punctual (an important signal of respect); doesn't get interrupted by phone calls during a consultation; radiates warmth, affirmation, optimism, and concern); listens attentively without impatient interruptions; poses open-ended questions, repeating and summarizing what has been said; doesn't use words that injure or maim; shows a readiness to acknowledge his or her errors; is sparing in use of procedures, refrains from multiple referrals to sub-specialists, and yet acknowledges his or her limitations, and finally, neither exaggerates minor illnesses nor is overwhelmed by major ones.

Other valuable characteristics of a good physician are a tolerance of uncertainty and a strong commitment to truth. "Paradoxically, taking uncertainty into account can enhance a physician's therapeutic effectiveness, because it demonstrates his honesty, his willingness to be more engaged with his patients, his commitment to the reality of the situation rather than resorting to evasion, half-truth, and even lies. And it makes it easier for the doctor to change course if the first strategy fails, to keep trying. Uncertainty sometimes is essential for success." (p.155, Groopman, 2008). Full disclosure of the truth generally benefits patients, although it is difficult to apply any simple set of rules in a medical context. General guidelines on truthfulness are unlikely ever to replace the physician's personal judgment of what a patient is willing to hear or able to understand.

In principle, it would seem possible for physicians to make peer ratings of the effectiveness of their colleagues, but this rarely happens in practice, except during examinations for various types of formal qualification, or following a determination of gross professional incompetence by a committee of the College of Physicians.

Chapter 7

MOTIVATORS, STRESSORS, JOB SATISFACTION AND PERSONAL QUALITIES OF A GOOD PHYSICIAN

The effectiveness of a doctor is likely to be enhanced if he or she is well-motivated, manages to minimize work-related stresses, finds his or her job satisfying, and has appropriate personal characteristics for the tasks that must be performed.

MOTIVATION

Few have attempted to measure the motivations of individual physicians, although this is likely to have an important bearing on the quality of the care that they offer. Too often, particularly in North America, the primary factors influencing behaviour appear to be hopes of a large income, attempts to avoid malpractice lawsuits, and an unwillingness to serve outside of normal office hours. Physicians may also be unwilling to concede their limitations as healers. Sometimes it is more appropriate to give palliative treatment rather than insist on heroic attempts to save a life. A good doctor recognizes that he or she is not omnipotent.

Motivations have been examined among university students. Kirkcaldy, Furnham & Lynn (1992) explored differences in work attitudes and occupational interests between 1000 UK and German students, British students showed a preference for business–oriented occupations, small business ownership or working as a company director. In contrast, German students frequently sought to become a doctor, social worker or teacher. Achievement motivation correlated significantly with occupations carrying social recognition (e.g. company director, doctor and/or teacher). A competitive work attitude was associated with a preference for occupations symbolizing success (business owner, director or physician). For the German students, interest in becoming a physician appeared related more to opportunities for competition and the work ethic than to attitudes towards money.

Odberg, Eriksen & Petersson (1995) explored the motivations of medical students, including their choice of speciality. The students' responses suggested they were both autonomy-oriented (seeking independence and rationality) and relation-oriented (sensitive in their relationships with others); they expected a doctor to be professionally competent and to relate effectively to his or her patients. The study did not disclose any gender differences either in perceived reasons for becoming a doctor or in the qualities making a good doctor, although female students were more likely to show an interest in interpersonal-oriented specialities, whereas men aimed for autonomy-oriented specialities. The authors argued that the increasing proportion of women entering the medical profession underlined the current shift towards less prestigious, interpersonal-oriented specialities, albeit at a price of a lower overall influence for the graduate.

Unfortunately, some medical school applicants may be motivated by a desire to help others as a means of coping with their own personal emotional and social inadequacies. Such candidates are unlikely to make good doctors. When the real demands of the profession emerge after completion of training, these individuals are prone to burnout and/or psychosomatic disorders. Another problem with some applicants is that well-intentioned but prestige-oriented parents may have channelled a child's interest into medicine – even though such a career does not fit the child's interests or personal strengths.

STRESSORS

Given the self-selection generally involved in career choices, it is difficult to compare levels of stress between professions. However, it is commonly accepted that many physicians find their profession stressful. Kirkcaldy, Athanasou and Trimpop (2000) used a repertory grid analysis to analyse sources of job-related stress among medical and paramedical professionals. Features that were identified included the personal context (family situation), the type of appointment (physician vs. assistant vs. paramedical), the form of social organisation (relationships with co-workers and/or boss), working conditions (salary, vacation provisions, etc.), any excessive workload, physical dangers (risks of infection and disease) and unpredictable events (time pressures, unexpected interruptions). In this analysis, a personal stress construct overlays any common meaning of the phenomenon (Tables 1 & 2).

Table I — Content analysis of some antecedent influences of stress in medical work settings.

Category	Antecedents
Work and organisational influences	Workload Excessive job demands Demands of the job Heavy workload Administrative overload Routine work Role-related demands Intense involvement over long periods of time Time pressures Constant time pressures Unpredictable interruptions Disruptive events Practice administration Staff conflicts Stress among colleagues Organisational climate and structure Stricter regulations Loss of autonomy Threat of malpractice suits Inadequate preparation Professional development. Working for College membership
Patient influences	Patients' unrealistic expectations Patients' expectations Coping with difficult patients Maintenance of empathic response with patients Existential dilemmas Dealing with dying and death Emotional involvement Confrontation with emotional suffering Feelings of helplessness
Personality influences	Specific personality types in medicine Situations that are emotionally demanding
Personal–family influences	Family–job conflicts Disruptions to social life Home–work interface Demands of work on family life Lack of leisure and free time Spillover problems in home and family life

Sources: Chambers et al;5 Constantini et al;7 Cooper et al;8 Harris;9 Makin et al;10 McCranie and Brandsma;11 Richardsen and Burke;12 Route and Route;13 Sutherland and Cooper;14,15 Symons and Persaud.16
Kirkcaldy, Athanasou & Trimpop (2000) with permission from Wiley and Sons.

Richardsen and Burke (1991) commented that for Canadian physicians "work pressures inherent in medical practice, disruptive events on the job may be stressful. Physicians are increasingly exposed to actual or threats of malpractice suits. After a malpractice suit, many physicians report feeling depressed and frustrated, they are less satisfied with their practice and start considering early retirement". They add "Doctors are often frustrated over loss of autonomy with stricter Medicare regulations, disillusioned over challenges to their competence by both professional boards and patients... (who are) becoming more knowledgeable consumers... and asking second opinions... the need for physicians to keep up their own level of medical knowledge is increasing" (p. 1179).

Table II — Supplementary table available on request. Some antecedents of stress in medical work settings.

Investigator	Antecedents
Chambers et al.[5]	Family–job conflicts Patients' unrealistic expectations Disruptions to social life Working for College membership
Constantini et al.[7]	Dealing with dying and death Feelings of helplessness Maintenance of empathic response with patients
Cooper et al.[8]	Excessive job demands Practice administration Patients' expectations
Harris[9]	Workload Staff conflicts Inadequate preparation Existential dilemmas
Makin et al.[10]	Unpredictable interruptions Administrative overload Routine work Emotional involvement Home–work interface
McCranie and Brandsma[11]	Intense involvement over long periods of time Situations that are emotionally demanding Confrontation with emotional suffering
Richardsen and Burke[12]	Disruptive events Threat of malpractice suits Loss of autonomy Stricter regulations Professional development
Rout and Rout[13]	Time pressures Demands of work on family life Coping with difficult patients
Sutherland and Cooper[14]	Heavy workload Constant time pressures Lack of leisure and free time Spillover problems in home and family life
Sutherland and Cooper[15]	Demands of the job Role-related demands Organisational climate and structure
Symons and Persaud[16]	Stress among colleagues Specific personality types in medicine

Reproduced with the permission of Wiley and Sons (Stress Medicine, Kirkcaldy, Athanasou & Trimpop, 2000) (upper numerals refer to reference number in original citation)

In a somewhat divergent opinion, Cooper, Rout and Faragher (1989) maintained that established general practitioners did not find either dealing with terminally ill patients or the need to maintain technical skills a source of occupational stress. In their view, job-related stress originated primarily through excessive job demands, the practical needs of practice administration, and patients' expectations. For GP registrars (British trainee family physicians, typically doctors with a young family) Chambers, Wall and Campbell, (1996) suggested that stress arose from family-job conflicts, disruption of social life, unrealistic patient expectations, the learning of unfamiliar tasks, and the need to study for Membership of the Royal College of GPs (a vast syllabus, plus a requirement to complete specific projects).

Comparing medical practitioners with para-medical personnel, Kirkcaldy, Brown, Furnham & Trimpop (2002) found that physicians were more stressed, but also reported higher rates of job satisfaction and more positive perception of their work environment than the paramedical staff. The length of working hours was the most significant stressor for medical personnel. Women generally expressed more favourable views than men. Whereas male paramedical personnel reported greater occupational stress than women, female doctors reported greater stress than their male counterparts.

JOB SATISFACTION

The various professions that contribute to comprehensive medical care all have an impact on a physician's job satisfaction. Kirkcaldy & Pope (1992) applied structural analysis to identify perceptions of "self" and "other" within a multidisciplinary medical hospital team. Physicians perceived themselves as separate from the psychological and therapeutic staff and patients' dependents. The patient was seen as falling within the network of the doctor's daily medical programmes and, although the psychological requirements of the patients were acknowledged, the physician applied "emotional distancing" as a way of coping with his or her task. The patient perceived the physician as more than a healer of the body (Kirkcaldy & Pope, 1992), investing in a high level of personal care, offering psychological support and providing important offers of well-being. Ray and Baum (1985) had previously observed that doctors are frequently questioned on social, psychological and ethical topics outside their domains of formal professional competency. Generally, physicians rely on their authority, without which it would be difficult to convince the patient to accept uncomfortable, distressing, painful and possibly incomprehensible treatment. The invested authority may help the patient too, bringing relief from a difficult decision-making process.

Pillay (2008) found that South African general practitioners were satisfied with the social and personal aspects of their work, but were likely to express dissatisfaction with the practice environment. Tension was experienced in complying with frequent patient requests and expectations such as the provision of medical reports, and absenteeism notes, and/or inappropriate demands for medication or surgery. Significant predictors of low work-satisfaction included being female, working in large groups, more than 20 years of practice, treating a high proportion of insured patients and dealing with "incentives" designed to preserve health-care resources. The greatest satisfaction was observed among those enjoying clinical freedom or with favourable perceptions of "managed" care, those remunerated on a fee-for-service basis and those working in small professional groups. The majority of Greek interns perceived their work as extremely stressful, and many reported a high degree of job dissatisfaction (Antoniou, Cooper & Davidson, 2008). Working hours of the interns were long and conditions were difficult during night shifts. Hospitals commonly lacked air-conditioning and staff rest quarters were noisy. Opportunities for social interaction were limited, and superiors provided little support or sympathy. Male doctors were also irritated by frequent patient complaints about their treatment and the quality of their hospital stay. Finally, adverse media publicity was compounded by a fear of making mistakes, and there was overall dissatisfaction with the moral and economic aspects of their work.

Some have argued that there is a need and an opportunity to learn by focussing on areas of dissatisfaction in a physician's practice. Peterkin (2009) listed ten major stressors for Canadian doctors: excessive workloads: frequent night calls; insufficient sleep (less than 3 hours some nights); uncompromising consultants; too much routine, tedious work and record-keeping; high death rates among patients; scarce contact with fellow colleagues; inadequate sexual activity, and high peer competition/rivalry. Bogue and colleagues (2006) identified as causes of dissatisfaction efforts at cost containment; a limited quantity and quality of personal time; insufficient opportunities for research and teaching; utilisation reviews (by hospitals); lack of autonomy; an inadequate income level; administrative responsibilities; a poor organisational climate; and an excessive workload. They also listed sources of job satisfaction: positive relationships with patients and colleagues; a successful resolution of family issues; opportunities for personal growth; freedom to provide quality care; availability of office and hospital resources, and the prestige of being a physician. They suggested that happiness among doctors focussed on their interactions with people, whether in their own families, in their organisation or practice, and in providing "intelligent" care for their patients. Interviews with physicians who expressed the highest levels of satisfaction led to the recommendation of several interventions: design of a "healthy" work environment (allowing personal choice in practice structure and organisation); exercising the body, enhancing diet and allowing adequate recuperation from potential stressors; promoting creative expression of the art of medicine; engagement with patients (improvement of personal listening skills, understanding and empowerment of patients); opportunities for travel (including cultural comparisons to assess the advantages of one's own medical care service); ensuring a clear demarcation between work and leisure/family time; and regulating emotional stress (identifying potential triggers and somatic cues).

Overall, job satisfaction seems likely when physicians, health care managers, administrators and social and health policy makers learn to cooperate with each other. Nevertheless, many physicians still seek less involvement of health care organisations and administrators in the decision-making process. Unfortunately, relationships between medical and administrative staff are frequently burdened by "power and role" struggles. In their daily tasks, doctors are required to adhere to the regulations imposed by their superiors as well as the time-intensive demands of administrative and organisational chores associated with economic constraints imposed by health insurance companies and hospital administrators. Constraints may include time limits for consultations and restrictions on the practitioner's decision-making with regard to treatment options. An additional "communication" pressure may be experienced, resulting from different priority ratings and personal stress-coping strategies. It seems clear that whereas a containment of the financial costs of health care is typically a central aim of administration, the "peripheral constraints" set by clinical management policies are often perceived as "irritating and random" by medical and allied personnel, and counter-productive to optimal patient treatment. Overall, the impression is often formed that physicians do not fully appreciate the economic limitations of any health care system; they have difficulty in reconciling the perceived needs of the individual patient with the impact of the proposed treatment upon the health care system as a whole. For the medical director and consultant physicians, the resulting role conflicts may cause them to become alienated from their personnel.

OPTIMAL PERSONAL CHARACTERISTICS

The optimal personal characteristics of a good doctor probably differ not only with specialty, but also between a solo practice and participation in a large, multi-disciplinary health team. Rudland & Mires (2005) had first year medical students complete a questionnaire on their perceptions of the general characteristics and backgrounds of doctors and nurses. Nurses were perceived as more caring and doctors as more arrogant. Nurses were seen as having lower academic ability, competence and status, but as sharing equivalent degrees of life experience. The authors argued that such impressions probably reflected societal stereotypes of the occupational role, status and responsibilities of physicians and nurses in contemporary medicine. Kirkcaldy, Pope and Siefen (1993) explored the diverse roles of medical health professionals in a child psychiatry clinic. Physicians were seen as powerful figures in the multidisciplinary team, especially with respect to decision-making and delegating. Social workers and psychologists were isolated from the rest of the treatment team and were more closely allied with the child's parents, perceiving the parents as highly influential and similar to the patient in their role. The physicians did not appear associated with either parents or patient; both physicians and nursing staff worked primarily through the hospital administration, and the administrative ties held a potential for role conflict.

Many studies to date have suggested that a good doctor needs interpersonal skills rather than academic brilliance. Particularly desirable characteristics are empathy and a willingness to listen. A longitudinal study of Flemish medical students (Lievens et al., 2002) found that conscientiousness (self-discipline and self-achievement) was a significant predictor of final pre-clinical year grades. Students who scored low on conscientiousness and high on gregariousness/affiliation and excitement seeking were unlikely to score well in their examinations. Nevertheless, characteristics of extraversion and agreeableness were important contributors to interpersonal skills, facilitating communication and collaborative efforts.

Chapter 8

ECONOMIC ASSESSMENTS OF THE QUALITY OF HEALTH CARE

Medical expenditures have soared in most Western industrialised nations for at least a couple of decades, to the alarm of politicians and health care administrators. Factors increasing costs include ever more sophisticated options in medical technology, an aging population, a desire to reduce inequities of health care, increased expectations of medical services among the population, and (recently) a rapid increase in the percentage of unemployed people (such individuals commonly adopt an adverse lifestyle and thus make heavy demands on medical systems). The problem of rising costs is further exacerbated by the current economic recession, leading to demands for a careful and detailed economic assessment of the effectiveness of all health care expenditures. Although some have questioned the ethics of a cost-benefit focussed approach, the hard fact remains that even in the richest of countries the potential to allow ever-more costly forms of treatment now exceeds the ability of those countries to provide such services on a universal basis. It is thus necessary to look very carefully at the efficacy of every proposed intervention, and to consider dispassionately for which population groups such treatment is appropriate, necessary and justified.

The financial aspects of health care and medical services are rarely discussed openly, either in the general social context or in reference to the reimbursement of doctors, nurses and hospitals. Nevertheless, some methods of payment for medical services provide incentives that encourage hospital administrators or individual doctors to adopt complicated treatment plans that are likely to bring economic benefits to an institution or a practice rather than to the reimbursing insurance system. In consequence, hospital admissions officers may demand a shortening of stay for patients that are less "lucrative," and individual physicians may refuse to see patients where the payments for consultations are low. Among the German Federal States, the financial aspects of hospital care – including the anticipated duration of inpatient stay - are often pre-determined by the hospital administration and health insurance companies. In order to deal more fairly with the diversity of physical ailments, the range of individual reactions to these ailments and the complexity of illness-related influences, more differentiated criteria of reimbursement seem necessary. Individual physicians also need the freedom to make honest choices between treatment options that currently offer differing material rewards to themselves or the hospital system. The complicated nature of existing "monetary keys" confounds any simple economic analysis of today's patterns of medical treatment.

International comparisons of health care typically have relied on such outcomes as infant mortality statistics, average overall life expectancy, and mortality from selected diseases, such data being related to the fraction of a nation's gross-national product that is expended on medical and health care. However, it is also possible to measure the success of physicians when undertaking specific tasks (Sinclair, Lawson & Burge, 2008; Ashworth, Medina & Morgan, 2008; UK Department of Health, 2003) - e.g. restoring an appropriate lifestyle, optimizing body mass index, establishing regular physical activity and a good diet, reducing the percentage of current smokers in their practice and maintaining an appropriate level of blood pressure in their patients. Other relevant statistics include the number of physicians and hospital beds per 1000 population, per capita expenditures on medication, and the cost-efficacy of various approaches to reducing the prevalence of selected risk factors (Sawicki & Bastian, 2008; OECD, 2007; Griffin, Fox, Rusky & Buxton, 2000).

Current evaluations in terms of infant mortality and overall life expectancy require critical reconsideration. For example, overall infant mortality statistics need adjusting to account for any "saving" of the lives of infants destined to have a poor quality of life, and any estimate of overall life-expectancy must also be adjusted to reflect an individual's disease-free or quality-adjusted life span (Shephard, 1996). Clearly, there are many major fallacies in most economic analyses of health-care systems. Firstly, medical care is often assumed to be uniform across a nation. In some European countries, this is largely true (although often the upper socio-economic strata are more successful in attaining access to "universal" care). In countries such as Germany, the uneven distribution of medical practitioners is an issue of increasing concern. For instance, the density of physicians is low in the New Federal States (former DDR), and in cities such as Hamburg practices have gravitated towards affluent areas of the city. In the

United States, the tendency for physicians and hospital beds to congregate in wealthy suburbs is even more marked, leaving large segments of the poorer members of society with little access and a much poorer quality of health care. Even for those Americans who have medical insurance, a variety of "plans" offer widely differing options and restrictions upon treatment. Thus, aggregate figures for the health of the entire population have little meaning for the health economist. In Canada, a scheme of provincially transferable universal health care theoretically provides a relative uniform pattern of treatment. In practice, this is generally true of Southern Canada, but the geographic immensity of the Canadian north inevitably leads to wide discrepancies in the patterns of care that are available; many small settlements across the tundra and on the arctic coast are served mainly by a nurse-practitioner, advised by a Tel-Sat communication with an urban hospital centre (Hild, 2004).

The World Health Report (2001) attempted to compare health services around the world. It quickly became clear that the expenditure of a large fraction of a nation's GDP or GNP did not guarantee a superior level of health care. Indeed, Germany and Switzerland (with expenditures > 10 percent of GDP) were ranked 25th and 20th respectively in terms of the overall effectiveness of their health care systems. Kirkcaldy (2009) further examined OECD data for some 26 nations. In 2005-2006, the total medical expenditures expressed as a percentage of GDP were not significantly related to either infant mortality or life expectancy at birth (although the latter correlation approached statistical significance, $r=0.38$, $n=26$, $p<0.06$). There was also no statistically significant correlation between medical expenditures and scores on the Veenhoven happiness scale ($r=0.33$, $n=24$, $p>0.05$). The limited nature of such correlations is perhaps not surprising, given that the expenditure of rather similar percentages of GDP can mask enormous differences in absolute expenditures from one country to another. A second series of analyses in which the countries were extended to include many non-OECD nations, revealed that health expenditure as a percentage of GDP for the year 2009 was significantly correlated with life expectancy at birth ($r=0.56$, $p<0.001$, $n=47$) and infant mortality ($r=-0.51$, $p<0.001$) as well as psychological health – defined by Veenhoven's happiness scale ($r=0.50$, <0.002). Again this may be evidence that for the mainly European and industrialised nations, spending "beyond" a certain level of health care may not manifest itself in "improved health".

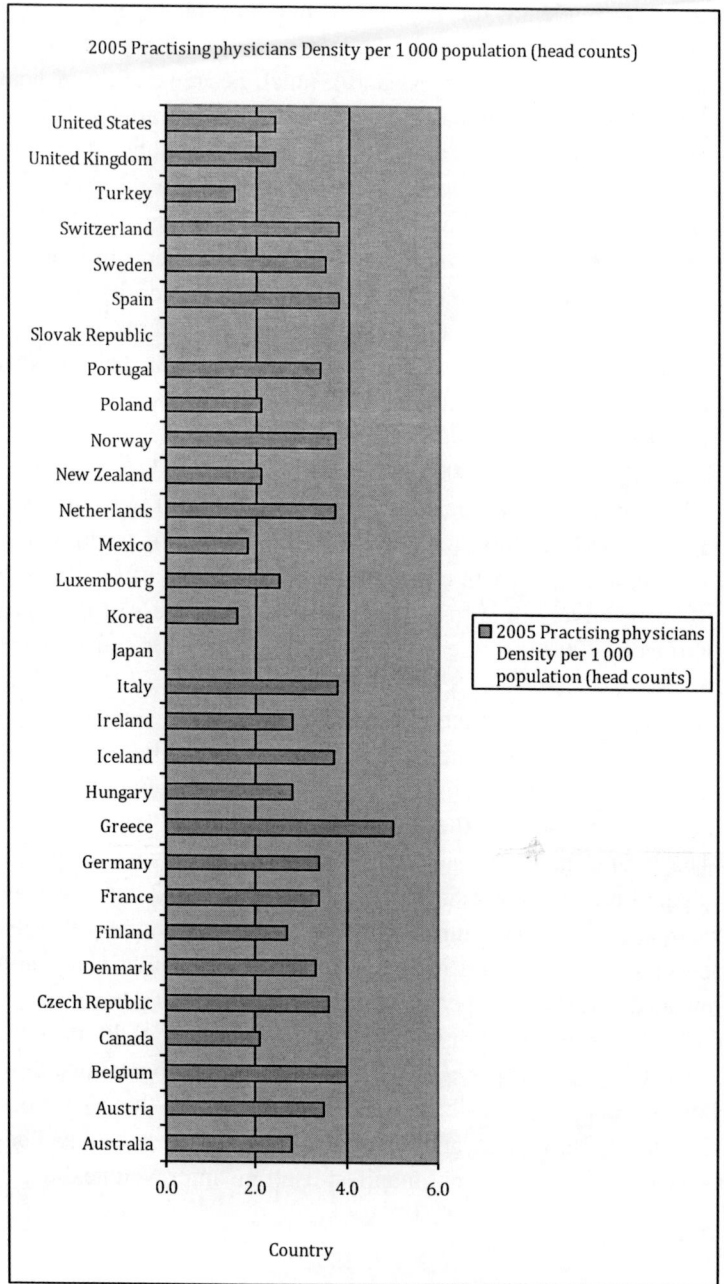

Figure 5. Number of Practising Physicians per 1000 population for countries in 2005 (drawn Kirkcaldy. Source: "OECD Health Data 2008, December 08, OECD, Paris"

The number of physicians per 1000 inhabitants (Figure 5) was greatest in Greece (4.9), followed by Belgium (4.0), Italy (3.8), Spain (3.8) and Switzerland (3.8). Among the countries surveyed, the lowest proportions of doctors were in Turkey (1.5), Korea (1.6), Mexico (1.8) and Japan (2.0). This index showed a weak relationship to life expectancy at birth (r=0.51, p<0.01) and infant mortality per 1000 births (r=-0.46, p<0.03), but was unrelated to psychological health/happiness (r=0.14, p>0.05). Weaknesses in this statistic contributing to the low coefficients of correlation include a poor distribution of physicians across both regions and specialties, and (in many countries) a lack of free universal access to practising physicians.

The percent of GDP spent on pharmaceutical products (2005) was not related to either life expectancy (-0.37, p>0.05) or infant mortality (r=0.12, p>0.05). In contrast, it was significantly correlated with happiness (but in the opposite direction to expectation, r=-0.58, p>0.005). There are problems of causality when interpreting this relationship; it may be that people in nations with a high prevalence of depression felt a need to spend more on medications, or it may be that spending on drugs did not counteract mental disorders. Unfortunately, resolution of this question is difficult, since available data often do not distinguish expenditures on psychopharmacologic agents from the purchase of other types of medication.

One of us recently compared the efficiency of medical expenditures by geographic region and the socio-political characteristics of selected countries (Figure 6). The groupings that were evaluated included: Scandinavian social democracies (Denmark, Finland, Norway & Sweden), European democracies (Belgium, France, Germany, Israel, Netherlands, Switzerland), South and Central American republics (Argentine, Brazil, Mexico, Nicaragua), North America (Canada and US) and poor tropical countries (Burkina Faso, Haiti, Cuba). Statistics for 2003-2008 published by WHO, 2003-2008 were reported as U.S. dollars per capita and percentages of GDP. The first statistic is somewhat susceptible to currency issues (for instance, apparently anomalous high medical expenditures in oil-rich Norway), and as noted above the second index is not very helpful, since the percentage of GDP allocated to medical programmes differs relatively little across countries, although a given absolute expenditure can buy much more in (say) Cuba than in a rich country such as Switzerland.

Selected outcomes for this analysis included life expectancy at birth (mean for men & women), healthy life expectancy (mean for men and women), adult mortality (both sexes) per 100,000, aged 15-60 years, years of disability (mean for both sexes), infant mortality per 1000 live births (male), maternal mortality per

100,000 live births, and cost ($) per year of healthy life expectancy. The analysis drew several main conclusions:

- the gross amount of medical expenditures had only a limited effect on outcomes, with the exception of maternal and infant mortality (where benefit was probably achieved through the control of infectious disease). In terms of overall life expectancy, the outcome appeared to plateau at an annual expenditure of around 1800 dollars per person, (Kirkcaldy & Siefen, 2005).
- medical expenditures in the poorest countries were so low that all indices of health were poorer than in other regions of the world.
- comparison of data for Canada and the U.S. showed that despite a harsh climate and a widely scattered population, the Canadian universal national health care system yielded substantially superior health outcomes than in the U.S., for about a half the cost of the private medical system favoured in the U.S.
- Cuba achieved similar outcomes to Canada on most indices, despite a tenth of the absolute expenditure, in part because it has a salaried medical service rather than a fee for service arrangement.

How far should policy decisions be influenced by such statistics? Lown (1999) has commented critically on the current concern with the financial aspects of health care. "The foremost objective of the system is cost containment, and to accomplish this, hospitals create vast bureaucracies of economic managers, accountants, and lawyers, now grown more numerous than the health care providers. Efficiency becomes the byword dictating homogenisation in dealing with any and all patient problems. Standard clinical guidelines and computer-driven algorithms define automatic courses of action for specified diagnostic categories" (p. 321, Lown, 1999).

Groopman (2008) has offered a further critique of the current micro-management approach adopted by many health economists, underlining that whilst electronic technology facilitates the organisation and accessibility of clinical information, the focus on "effectiveness" may "drive a wedge" into the physician-patient relationship. It may also increase cognitive errors, since the physician is directed to complete blanks on a template. An absence of open-ended questioning may discourage exploration of data that do not fit this template. Groopman argues that quality primary care demands a broader thinking style. "Any and every problem of human biology can present itself; it means making judicious decisions with limited data about children and adults, neither overreacting nor being blasé; it means wielding one's words with precision and with a profound appreciation of the social context of the patients" (p.100).

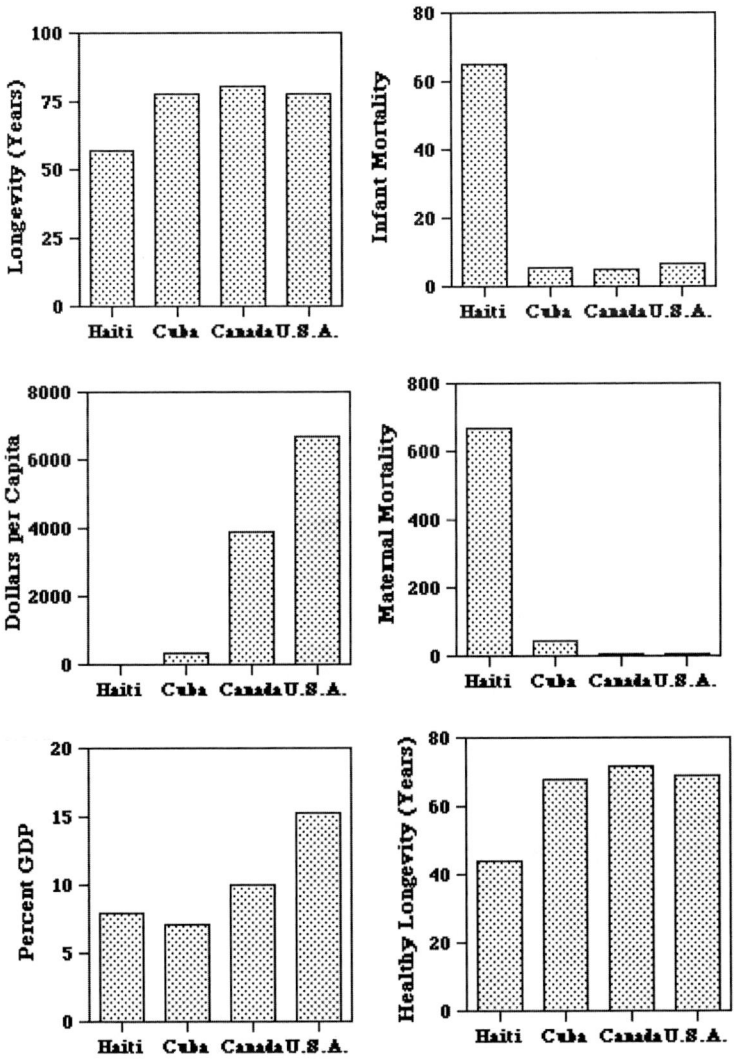

Figure 6. Selected health outcomes (longevity, healthy longevity, infant mortality, maternal mortality, dollar expenditures per capita and percent of GDP) for one poor country (Haiti), one country with a salaried health service (Cuba), one developed country with a universal fee-for-service system (Canada), and one country with private medical coverage (U.S.A.).

POLICY IMPLICATIONS FOR MEDICAL EDUCATION, CARE OF THE PHYSICIAN AND HEALTH SERVICE MANAGEMENT

The above review of the various factors affecting patient health, interactions between the patient and his or her physician, and resulting costs of medical services points to a need for early changes in several areas of policy and practice. Areas needing further consideration include the selection and training of medical students, plans for the continuing education and health maintenance of established physician, and decisions on overall medical care expenditures and methods of reimbursement.

Chapter 9

SELECTION AND TRAINING OF MEDICAL STUDENTS

SELECTION CRITERIA

In most countries, the selection of students for medical school is highly competitive. In the U.K., there are 40,000 applicants for some 5000 places (Ferguson, James & Madeley, 2002), and in Germany, 28,663 applicants vie for 8320 places. German dental schools also have 4507 candidates for a total of 1398 places, and Departments of Psychology report 14600 applicants for 3767 places. These figures suggest that medicine and the allied professions are popular educational goals, despite current stressors and uncertainties regarding future employment prospects.

Women are increasingly gravitating towards medicine as a career. By 2003-4, the number of applicants to U.S. medical school was higher for women (50.8%) than for men (Zelnio, 2009). Women were not admitted to London Medical Schools (except the "Royal Free Hospital") until 1947. The proportion of female medical students in the U.K. increased steadily from 20-25% in 1968 to > 50% by 1991. By 2002, 60.8% of students accepted to British medical or dental schools were women (Royal College of Physicians, 2006). In Germany, the proportion of female medical students rose from 46% to 59% between 1994 and 2004 and by 2006 56% of newly registered physicians were women (Forum Gesundheitspolitik, 2009). Female physicians were a rarity early in the 20th century, but by 1980, the figures were 17% for US, 19% for Germany, 20% France and 32% (medical doctors and dentists) in Israel (Compton Interactive Encyclopaedia, 2005). Interestingly, female physicians generally show some of the characteristics commonly lacking in male doctors, seeing fewer patients per day, but investing more time in talking to individual patients.

The selection of medical students still places a very strong emphasis on the academic attainments of candidates, although there is little objective evidence that this influences ultimate competence. McManus (1982) found scant proof that high grades in the United Kingdom's A-level school-leaving/University entrance qualifying examinations were associated either with success in pre-clinical and clinical courses, or with superior ability in the subsequent practise of medicine. A review of diverse studies showed correlations of only 0.10-0.25 between A level performance and success in medical school. On the other hand, there has also been little empirical validation of the specific personal and cognitive skills generally regarded as necessary for success in medicine.

Given the high demand for places in medical school, there is substantial opportunity to explore the motivation of potential medical students, to identify appropriate academic traits and personality types, and to recognise and exclude applicants who seem less likely to complete their studies for lack of motivation and/or ability. Nevertheless, it is easier to specify the ideal characteristics of a graduate than to indicate optimal methods of selection and training to meet these desiderata (Hurwitz & Vass, 2002). Plainly, in a task as individualistic as medical practice, much depends on intrinsic motivation and job satisfaction; after qualification the practitioner must often face a heavy workload in an isolated community, and resultant problems of substance abuse too often need correcting (BMJ Editor, 2008).

CURRICULUM

There are substantial cultural differences between countries in terms of both methods of medical teaching and ultimate clinical practice. Patterns of training differ widely between the UK (where practical learning on the hospital wards and role modelling are emphasized) (Cruess, Cruess & Steinert, 2008) and North America, where there is a heavy emphasis on book learning and classroom lectures, with very little direct contact between the student and the patient. The traditional teaching of medical students has emphasised patient evaluation as proceeding "in a discrete, linear way.. only after all the data are compiled should you formulate hypotheses about what might go wrong. These hypotheses should be winnowed by assigning statistical probabilities .... to each symptom, physical abnormality, and laboratory test: then you calculate the likely diagnosis. This is Bayesian analysis, a method of decision-making favoured by those who construct algorithms and strictly adhere to evidence-based practice. But, in fact, few if any physicians work with this mathematical paradigm." (Groopman, 2008, p. 11)

In most countries, the medical curriculum, needs expanding in many areas, to include an inculcation of sensitivity to anthropological and cultural issues, the development of personal and listening skills, instruction in elementary psychology and the techniques of implementing behavioural change, and the learning of practical procedures for the intelligent and effective prescription of physical activity, diet and other aspects of personal lifestyle.

In most systems, hospital specialists play a major part in the instruction of medical students, although there is little agreement as to whether this is particularly helpful to the learning process. Senior staff generally embody status and responsibility; they are likely to spend time teaching - in North America by lecturing, and in the European system by outpatient clinics and conducting ward-rounds that underline the doctor-patient relationship and the psychosocial features of medical care. Some observers view the lofty status and the dominant role modelling of the traditional teaching-hospital specialist as crucial to the inculcation of professional values, attitudes and behaviours among both medical students and junior doctors. However, Paice and colleagues (2002) found that medical students and young interns sought in their ideal role models attributes of interest/enthusiasm, favourable attitudes towards junior colleagues, compassion, integrity, openness and good relationships with patients - qualities more commonly found in a resident than in an established specialist.

DEVELOPMENT OF PERSONAL ATTRIBUTES

A sound academic base is certainly important to the implementation of evidence-based medical treatment, but the present review suggests the importance of giving at least equal weight to the development of appropriate personal attributes - a tolerance of stress, well-honed social skills, empathy with the patient, an ability to listen attentively and an ability to communicate the desired treatment plan concisely and effectively.

The medical school that one of us attended (RS) made an empiric test of the student's tolerance for long hours of work by requiring its ward clerks to work and study 21 hours per day for one week in four; this rather brutal approach certainly served to eliminate the faint of heart, Clode (2004) underlined the need for individuals able to tolerate stress in an Australian report entitled "The Conspiracy of Silence: Emotional Health among Medical Practitioners". He specified three factors that he perceived as currently contributing to stress among physicians: (i) personality characteristics − individuals gravitating towards the medical profession are likely to be workaholics, achievement oriented (with a need for social recognition) and emotionally sensitive, attributes that increase their risk of emotional ill—health, (ii) job-related stressors − direct (and often sole) responsibility for patient care and treatment outcomes; self-employment (a fee for service arrangement, with personal remuneration dependent upon this); and the pressures of the need to continue learning about new developments in medicine, and (iii) the current orientation of medical training, with its strong emphasis of academic excellence, inadequate social support of the student and a lack of emphasis on the development of social skills and the ability to communicate.

Some of the traditional expectations of the medical profession such as endurance of long working hours, and a willingness to make home visits at all hours of the day and night are perceived as less acceptable by the younger generation of doctors. Especially in German hospitals, there is now a growing desire to establish not only the traditional medical associations and colleges, but also union-organised medical groups; indeed, there have been a number of strikes where interns have demanded much shorter and more regular hours of work. **Moreover, there has clearly been a "feminisation" of the medical occupation** in recent years, with many more women now gravitating to medical professions. Often, these women are trying to integrate the demands of their occupation with the equally pressing needs of caring for young families. Moreover, these changes in the profile of contemporary medical practitioners is not restricted to women; increasing numbers of male doctors also try to integrate and reconcile the claims of family, work and recreation.

Aswani (2001) explored factors helpful in developing the capacity of students for empathy. Suggestions included a liberal and humanistic education, with exposure to literature and philosophy; specific training in interpersonal and communication skills; participation in workshops and seminars on the arts of attentive listening, sensitivity, and empathy; and even practical experience of being a patient − whether real or simulated - within the current system. The optimal practice of medicine certainly demands vivid creative skills, as exemplified in artistic expression and writing; such a talent seems of particular importance in developing social skills and compassion. In 1936, Freud was nominated for a Nobel Prize in literature, and he eventually received the Goethe Prize for his contribution to German writing. A long list of other noted physicians have also been outstanding authors, from classic writers such as Friedrich Schiller, Georg Büchner, Ludwig Büchner, Viktor Frankl, Mikhail Bulgarov, Anton Chekhov, Sir Arthur Conan Doyle, John Keats, and Erasmus Darwin to more contemporary writers such as W. Somerset Maugham, Oliver Sacks, Irvon Yalom, and Jerome Groopman. "While it has long been understood that clinical practice influenced the youthful writing of doctor-authors like Chekhov and William Carlos William, there is now emerging evidence that exposure to literature and writing during residency training can influence how young doctors approach their clinical work. By bringing short stories, poems and essays into hospital wards and medical schools, educators hope to encourage fresh thinking and help break down the wall between doctors and patients" (P.W. Chen, 2008).

Some medical schools have attempted to incorporate narrative competence into their curriculum, teaching practitioners to "acknowledge, absorb, interpret, and act on the stories and plights of others" (Charon, 2001, p. 1897). Charon suggested "understand(ing) the meaning and significance of stories through cognitive, symbolic and affective means ... (providing) a rich, resonant comprehension of a singular person's situation as it unfolds in time, whether in such texts as novels, newspaper stories, movies, and scripture or in such life setting as courtrooms, battlefields, marriages, and illnesses" (p. 1898). "Narrative medicine is clinical practise fortified with the knowledge of what to do with stories.... instead of exhorting clinicians to be professional, humanistic, empathetic and altruistic, we would rather offer them the narrative skills... to *convey* the professionalism, humanism, empathy and altruism that they possessed. And so we train clinicians, scholars, writers and patients, in the complex tasks of giving and receiving accounts of self. The most directive way to date to develop these skills is rigorous training in close reading and reflective writing" (Charon, 2009)

Newton and colleagues (2008) assessed the emotional empathy of students at the onset of each year of medical studies. Students who ultimately selected core careers (internal medicine, family medicine, obstetrics-gynaecology, paediatrics and psychiatry) showed higher empathy scores than those who found their vocation in other specialities. Vicarious empathy decreased significantly over the course of medical education. The authors were concerned by this apparent "hardening of the heart," since they judged compassion and concern as essential to a favourable doctor-patient relationship. They suggested that factors reducing empathy were the stress and anxiety resulting from a desire to overachieve in examinations, and media portrayal of physicians as idols, thus skewing the medical student's image of an ideal doctor.

Rinpoche & Shlim (2006) offered the following comments on developing compassion in the medical profession: "Patience is like an armour, and the stronger your compassion, the stronger the armour.... When insight is present, you don't become weary or discouraged. Your compassion needs to be suffused with this intelligent quality of seeing clearly. Otherwise, when you are confronted with people who don't want to listen to you, even when you've tried your best to be kind and caring, you may feel discouraged." (pp.135-136, Rinpoche & Shlim, 2006).

CARE OF THE PHYSICIAN

A good physician will plainly monitor and enhance his or her personal health, take measures to keep abreast of recent developments in medical knowledge, seek to enhance his or her people skills and show appropriate attitudes towards the management of risk in his or her life.

Chapter 10

MONITORING AND MAINTENANCE OF PERSONAL HEALTH

"By medicine life may be prolonged, yet death will seize the doctor too" (W. Shakespeare).

Medicine is oriented towards delaying death, but all (including the physician) are liable to illness and must ultimately die. It seems axiomatic that if a doctor is to practice effectively, he or she should seek to maintain good personal health; a clear example of an optimal lifestyle must be provided to those who seek the advice of the practitioner. However, this is too rarely the case.

As discussed above, the anxieties and uncertainties of medical practice expose the physician to a level of stress that is rarely encountered in many other occupations. Doctors and other members of the "helping professions" seem particularly prone to develop "burnout." McCranie and Brandsma (1988) described a "state of physical, emotional and mental exhaustion that occurs as a result of intense involvement .... in situations that are emotionally demanding. It is characterised in its extreme form by physical depletion and chronic fatigue, feelings of helplessness and hopelessness, and the development of negative attitudes towards self, work, life and other people" (p.30). The prevalence of burn-out among health professionals reflects the need to confront the emotional aspects of human suffering. Costantini, Solano, Di Napoli and Bosco, (1997) have argued that certain specialties "such as oncology and AIDS care, expose ... staff to higher work-related stress. The need to deal with dying and death, the feeling of helplessness, ... the limits of medicine in these pathologies, the length of the disease, the need to maintain an empathic reaction.... the risk that empathy might lead to identification, are potentially stressful ... for caregivers" (p 79).

Rinpoche & Shlim (2006) asserted "Doctors ... need to distance themselves from the pain, loneliness, and fear that many patients are suffering. If they identify too closely with their patients, they run the risk of emotional exhaustion. Emotional exhaustion can interfere with their ability to make clear decisions, so they try to maintain an objective distance, a distance that the patient interprets as not caring enough... the only way they feel they can care more for patients is by not caring too much." (p. 4, Rinpoche & Shlim, 2006).

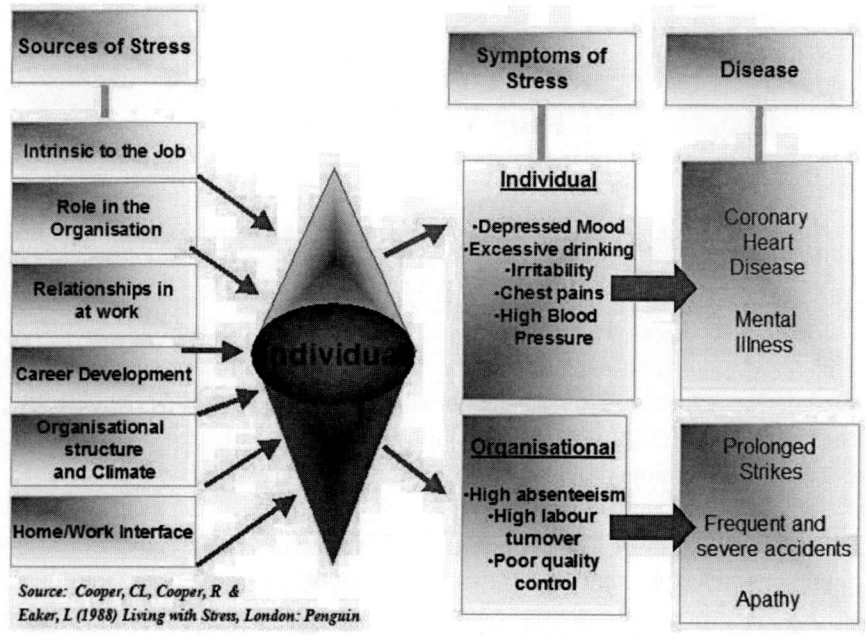

Figure 7. Transactional model of stress (Source: Cooper et al, 1988. With permission)

Too often, emotional involvement with the problems of their patients takes its toll on the health of physicians. Although they may enjoy better physical health than the general population, they have poorer psychological health, as shown by a high incidence of psychiatric disorders, drug and alcohol use, and suicide (Guthrie & Black, 1997). Sutherland and Cooper (1993) examined predictors of mental ill-health and job dissatisfaction among a representative sample of almost one thousand British general practitioners. Three major stressors were identified: *demands of the job and patients' expectations* (e.g. fear of assault, adverse publicity from the media, patients' complaints), *role-related demands* (e.g.

conflicts between their task and role demands, role ambiguity, serious implications of mistakes), and *organisational climate/structure* (the need to complete mundane administrative work, inadequate resources, low morale, staff shortages, lack of opportunities for consultation and communication). The extent of the doctor's social support network was a major determinant of job satisfaction. The authors suggested dealing with these stressors through a combination of individually focussed interventions such as time management and assertiveness training, cognitive restructuring, and the provision of opportunities for physical activity or relaxation, plus organisationally-oriented methods.

The transactional model is one of the most frequently cited representations of stress and its potential impact on physical and psychological health. Kirkcaldy and colleagues adopted this model in diverse studies aimed at identifying general and specific sources of work-related stress and their influence on various measures of health outcome. More particularly, they wanted to explore what individual variables were effective in reducing the possibly adverse effects of pressures associated with work.

In one such study, Kirkcaldy & Siefen (2002) compared the medical directors of German clinics with other groups with managerial responsibilities. Medical professionals tended to display greater job-related stress, specifically in relationship to workload, managerial role and daily hassles. Conversely, they indicated less stress relating to recognition and achievement than their peers in other professions. There were no inter-group differences in terms of Type A behaviour or patterns of coping, but senior physicians exhibited high scores for an internal locus of control. Most physicians evaluated their working environment positively. They were also likely to express intrinsic work satisfaction, organizational satisfaction and organizational security. The extent of daily hassles (day to day irritants and aggravations within the workplace) emerged as the single main predictor of physical and psychological health problems for this particular group of physicians.

Kirkcaldy & Siefen (1991) noted that relative to their female peers, male health care professionals in a large hospital were more inclined to report stress, complaining about relationships with their colleagues and finding a greater adverse impact of job pressures in their family lives. However, this difference may reflect in part a sex difference in the choice of specialty, since female physicians tend to opt for those types of practice where freer time schedules are possible.

In a more recent large-scale study, Kirkcaldy, Trimpop & Martin (2009) found that relative to others in ancillary professions, medical doctors were more likely to experience stress in their work, but they also reported higher satisfaction scores. The comparison between GPs and specialists (Figure 8) revealed that specialists were significantly more likely to show work-related stress and reported poorer work-place climates. Hence, job status would appear to exert a role in the subjective experience of stress among medical professionals.

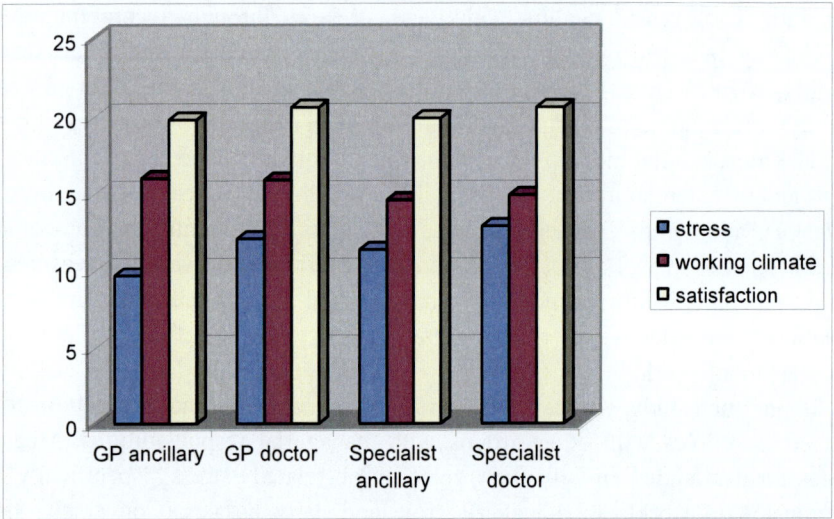

Figure 8. Differences in reported work stress and satisfaction with the work-place climate between ancillary personnel, general practitioners and specialist medical consultants

Symons and Persuade (1995) have suggested that most studies of stress focus excessively on the externals of medical practice such as hours and conditions of work, to the neglect of less comfortable questions such as "stress among colleagues" and the "gravitation of specific personality types" towards the medical profession, both of which seem to be significant issues contributing to manifestations of stress.

ADVERSE CONSEQUENCES OF STRESS

Many doctors like to perceive themselves as invincible. Thus, A'Brook (1990) noted the reluctance of doctors to disclose personal problems such as psychotic or depressive illnesses and the development of chemical dependencies. Nevertheless, in response to direct questioning, Fuchs (2008) noted that 39% of female doctors admitted to experiencing depression, compared with 30% of other females who had earned doctoral degrees. Psychiatric conditions common among physicians include major depression, ethanol and drug abuse, bipolar disorder, anxiety disorder and various other personality disorders (Fung, 2007). Schattner & Colman (1998) found that at any one time the scores on 13% of questionnaires completed physicians indicated a severe psychiatric disturbance. The reported underlying stressors included threats of litigation; work overload, insufficient earnings; interactions with difficult patients, and administrative/paperwork demands; with the probable exception of an inadequate income, all of these seem plausible and legitimate concerns.

Health statistics confirm the potentially deleterious effects of stressors on health-care professionals. Thus in their middle years, (female) nurses had a shorter life-expectancy than other female-dominated occupations such as social workers, secretaries, and teachers (Elliot and Eisdorfer, 1982). Likewise, British physicians had an increased risk of dying from suicide, hepatic cirrhosis, accidental poisoning and accidents in general (Registrar General, 1978). Various other authors have noted high levels of psychiatric illness among (male) doctors (Murray, 1977), borderline depression or depressive bouts (Caplan, 1994), sustained emotional distress among junior doctors (Cartwright, 1987), elevated job-related anxiety and depression (Rucinski and Cybulska, 1985; Belfer, 1989), greater alcohol dependence (up to seven times more for doctors than for control groups of similar social class) (Brooke, Edwards and Taylor, 1991; Bissel, 1976) and a high proportion of physicians who smoked and drank to excess (Allibone et al.; 1981).

Too frequently, psychiatric disturbances are sufficiently severe to precipitate suicide. Lindeman and coworkers (1996) compared the suicide rates of British physicians with those of the general population; figures were 1.1-3.4 times higher for male and 2.5-5.7 times higher for female doctors. Risks relative to other professionals were also 1.5-3.8 higher for male and 3.7-4.5 higher for female physicians. Likewise, suicide rates for physicians in the U.S. were higher than in all other professional groups (males 70%, females 40% higher than the general population). Shernhammer & Colditz (2004) reviewed 25 U.S. studies; suicide rates relative to the general population were 40 percent higher for males and 130 percent higher for females, although these authors cautioned that there was a possible publication bias.

These various statistics emphasize the need for an effective physician to conserve both physical and mental health. A good physician recognizes the potential danger to others from continued self-medication and an unwillingness to admit personal illness. The Australian Medical Association (2006) has examined practical preventive and therapeutic options for physicians. Suggestions included:

maintaining a good relationship with a trusting fellow physician and developing a network of peers to allow "debriefing, support and mentorship," providing practitioners with relevant information on stress factors in their professional and personal lives, and offering peer assistance to those showing manifestations of stress. The Australian report also underlined the health importance of taking regular vacations, developing an awareness of personal nutrition and taking time out for family and lifestyle pursuits, whether as medical students or qualified practitioners.

Maintaining a Current Knowledge Base

The half-life of medical knowledge is getting shorter year by year and the attempts of a busy practitioner to maintain a current knowledge base may lead to disappointment and exhaustion. The good physician must maintain competence in both the "manual and technical" aspects of the trade. Financial pressures impose time constraints that limit opportunities for further learning, and the pursuit of such instruction is liable to cause conflicts with more or less competitive colleagues. Groups such as Colleges of General Practitioners have developed credit systems that encourage physicians to keep up to date with recent advances in medicine. However, many such systems are voluntary, and sometimes course credit can be obtained simply by staying at a conference hotel without actually listening to the lectures. Further, the content of many courses is biased because of sponsorship by multinational drug companies, and accessory reading may be provided by drug company detail representatives rather than by reprints from peer-reviewed and objective scientific journals.

Development of Personal Skills

Many of the reports reviewed above underline the need to develop the personal and interactive skills of doctors as a part of their continuing education. "Sick people need physicians who can understand their diseases, treat their medical problems, and accompany them through their illnesses. Despite medicine's recent dazzling technological progress.... physicians sometimes lack the capacities to recognise the plights of their patients, to extend empathy towards those who suffer, and to join honestly and courageously with patients in their illnesses" (Charon, 2001, p. 1987).

DEALING WITH UNCERTAINTY

In a review study. Hayward (2006) comments on the needs a doctor's education must address, particularly the anxieties (both rational and irrational) associated with the uncertainties in decisions, which impact on life and death. He asserts "Irrationality ensures that the perception by individuals of their state of health (and the estimation of this by their doctor) can never be certain or, in a scientific sense, entirely predictable; therefore, the effects of treatment must always be, to some extent, uncertain (and unpredictable) as well. At the same time, uncertainty inevitably contributes to the element of irrationality that invests the relationship between doctor and patient" (p. 74/75). There are probably few occupations that entail such a high degree of "doubt" and yet expect such a high degree of confidence and self-assurance. Perhaps this indispensable quality of sceptical empiricism among the medical profession is what Tabel (2007) meant when he suggests "A theory is like medicine ... often useless, sometimes necessary, always self-serving, and on occasion lethal. So it needs to be used with care, moderation, and close cooperation" (p.285). Decision-making processes are not as unambiguous and straightforward as we would wish, so that "Nowhere is the equation, condition A, if followed by treatment B, will produce result C, less certain than in the practice of clinical medicine. Yet major decisions affecting life and death need to be made against such a background. The diagnosis of condition A can be wrong because the evidence upon which it is based is insufficient or misleading, or because of human error. The patient may have other (sometimes occult) conditions that will clash in unpredictable ways with treatment B. Treatment B may have other effects in addition to producing result C and these may interfere with its predicted effects on condition A. Finally, the interplay between the personality of the doctor and the personality of the patient may alter the perception (by either the doctor, or the patient, or both) that result C has been achieved at all. Such uncertainty can be as dispiriting for doctors as it is for patients, often leading to denial (by both parties) that such uncertainty even exists" (Hayward, 2006, p. 75).

MANAGEMENT OF RISKS AND ERRORS

Given the imprecise nature of medicine, occasional errors of diagnosis and judgment are inevitable. Just over a half of respondents in a European Union study (EU, 2006) suggested that hospital patients could help in avoiding medical mistakes. The majority of respondents in Denmark (70%), Hungary (66%), Slovenia (62%) and Finland (61%) believed that a patient could influence the quality of treatment. Expectations of preventing hospital errors were lower for Germans (17%), Austrians (17%), Estonians (21%) and Portuguese (23%), with 38% of Germans, 23% of Portuguese and 25% of Austrians thinking this "not at all likely."

The risks of an adverse outcome differ to some extent with speciality. Critical incidents are common in surgery (Cooper et al, 2002) and obstetrics. Ennis and Vincent (1990) listed three major concerns in childbirth - insufficient foetal heart monitoring, inadequate supervision from more senior medical personnel, and mismanagement when delivering by forceps.

Nevertheless, a good physician can be identified by his or her attitudes to the management of both risks and errors. Some have argued that patient demands for shortened waiting times and more rapid decision-making are in themselves predisposed to errors. One way a physician can reduce error is to take more time on a given procedure. Doctors in primary care – paediatricians, general practitioners and/or internists – typically earn lower incomes than specialists. Groopman (2008) has argued that if a primary care physician spends an hour trying to reach a diagnosis then the resulting payment is meagre. "Many doctors have reacted by truncating visits to ten or fifteen minutes.... working in haste can not only increase cognitive mistakes but impair ...communication of ... basic information about treatment." (p. 86). In a study of 900 patients, Groopman found that two-thirds of physicians failed to inform the patient either how long he or she should take a new medication, or of potential side-effects; indeed, almost a half of doctors did not seem to have specified either dosage or duration of treatment.

Patient expectations of infallibility and an unrealistic belief in the capacity for instantaneous diagnosis may also contribute to mistakes. Banja (2007) has drawn attention to a culture of medical narcissism... "a psychological defence whose function is to protect the professional from an assault on his or her sense of self... (and) in the instance of medical error, one's natural, self-protective inclination is to conceal or obfuscate the error for fear that its disclosure will eventuate in malpractice litigation... the very thought of disclosing the error is so fraught with embarrassment, anxiety, and humiliation, that it is easy to understand why health professionals might look for reasons to excuse their moral obligation to disclose it or will conduct the communication in a non-incriminating way."

In the past, physicians often resisted admitting mistakes in diagnosis and treatment because of fears of litigation. Doctors also believed that admitting a mistake would perforate their aura of "infallibility and omniscience," which some have judged as crucial to patient confidence and compliance. However, this seems a false premise, since a failure to admit mistakes gives an air of arrogance and unkindness. Tavris and Aronson (2007) have commented on a recent shift in thinking, with physicians and clinics now encouraged to divulge and where possible to correct medical errors. Patients seem less likely to take legal action if a mistake is admitted and an appropriate apology offered.

IMPLICATIONS FOR HEALTH SERVICE MANAGEMENT

Deciding on an appropriate level of national expenditure on preventive medicine and health care, and the devising of optimal methods for the reimbursement of various categories of service remain key issues for the health economist to resolve. An increase in medical expenditures does not necessarily result in a delivery of superior health care. In theory, adjustments to methods of physician and hospital reimbursement might improve patterns of medical practice and health care delivery, although to date the treatment options selected have shown little apparent relationship to methods of payment (Kuusela, Variomki, Hinka & Rautava, 2004).

Payment for services rendered (the model commonly adopted in the US and Canada) has the major disadvantage of encouraging over-treatment (e.g. frequent office visits for weighing of the obese, and the frequent measuring of casual blood pressures in supposedly hypertensive patients). The UK system that makes annual payments per patient enrolled is theoretically good if sufficient doctors are available to allow patients a choice of practitioner. But in practice, such a system may lead to over-consultation by the patient and attempts by the doctor to empty a crowded surgery by hasty and sometimes unnecessary prescriptions. Other European health care systems such as that established in Germany afford easy and quick access to treatment, but seem rather costly. One recent option is to establish norms of prescription and procedures relative to practice as a whole and the age and sex of the patient. This type of plan is operated by some Health Maintenance Organizations in the US, and in the UK there have been plans to allow a given doctor a pool of W dollars for investigations, X dollars to spend on drugs, Y to spend on hospital referrals and Z for surgical treatments. In theory, this could minimize unnecessary treatments, although there remains at least a theoretical danger that a doctor or an HMO could by-pass controls by accepting only low maintenance patients.

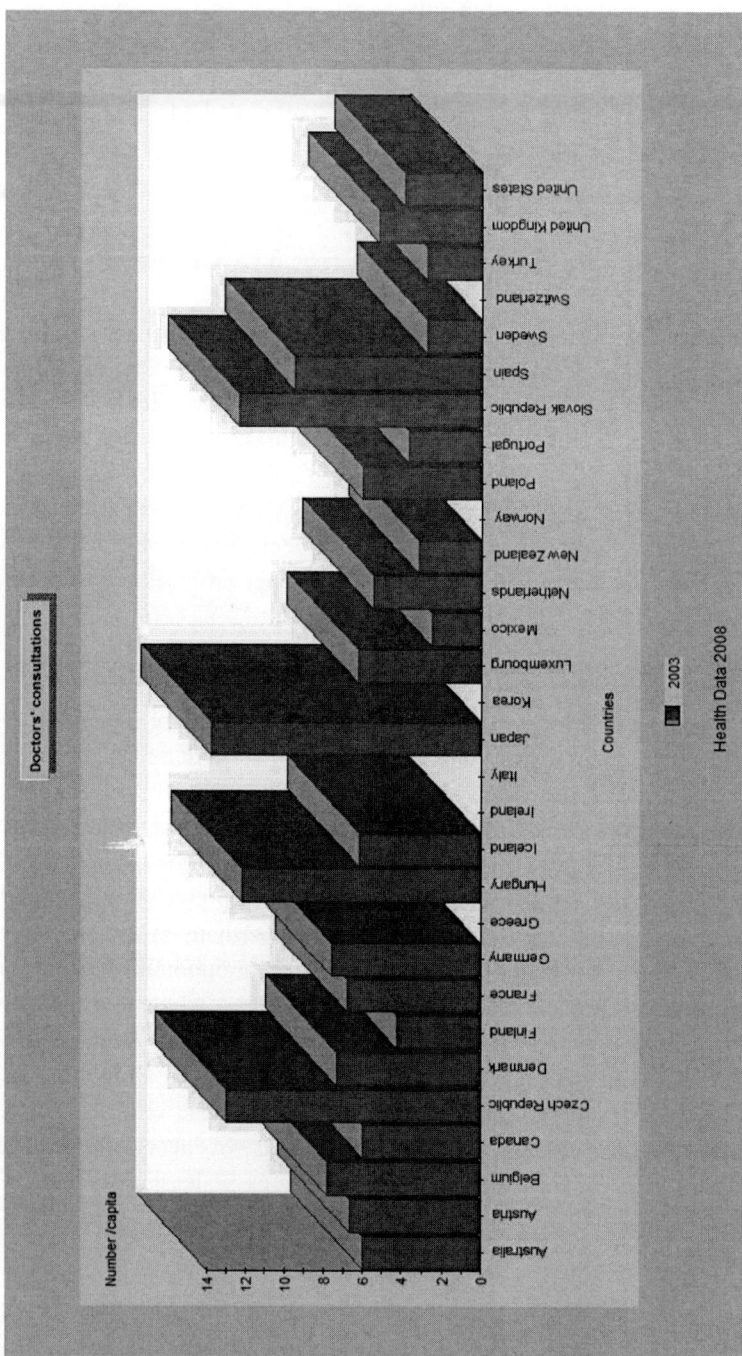

Figure 9. Frequency of medical consultations across nations (Source OECD Data 2003. Data missing for Greece, Ireland, Italy, Korea, Norway and Switzerland)

For economic reasons it might be useful to ration care by setting specific age limits at which definitive treatment should be replaced by palliative care - for example, one could allow an expenditure of a specified sum IF the resulting treatment gave the patient one additional year of quality-adjusted lifespan (this year is commonly equated to a sum of $20,000-100,000 dollars). Finally, modest user fees may have their place in setting an appropriate level of treatment and deterring excessive demands from patients.

The figure 9 reveals that nations such as USA, Germany and Luxemburg, which invest a significantly larger amount of money into medical care relative to other countries, do not necessarily see more frequent visits to physicians. It seems likely that costs incurred in these medical systems are related less to the number of doctor visits and more to the use of costly medical diagnostic tests and complicated surgical interventions.

An examination of the above figure reveals that physician consultations are more frequent in some nations (e.g. Japan, Czech Republic, Hungary and the Slovak Republic) than in others. Nations with low rates of consultations include Mexico, Turkey, Sweden and New Zealand. What explanations can be offered for these differential rates of medical dialogue? Are nations exhibiting higher rates of consultation less healthy, or indeed as a result of frequent visits and prompt confrontation with an ailment, are they healthier? Does the frequency of consulting a medical doctor reflect differing cultural beliefs concerning traditional medical care? Or do other socio-economic factors play a role in determining whether or not a doctor is sought to treat an illness? The OECD – in their 2003 date base – made efforts to produce a measure of medical consultations allowing comparisons across nations, while admitting that it is a basic measure of the magnitude of the services, taking the overall number of physician contacts. This in turn will depend on the availability of doctors (density per 1000 of the population) and the costs of consultation to the individual. Germany, Greece and France are among those nations allowing direct contact with a medical specialist, and others such as the United Kingdom, Netherlands and Austria require approaching a **"gatekeeper" first in the form of a general practitioner**, which presumably would increase (or decrease) frequency of medical visits. In the UK consultations do not include visits to specialist from the independent sector – and in Portugal and Turkey visits to private practitioners are excluded – nor does it include consultations on the NHS direct line, for services by phone. The US statistic, in contrast includes prescriptions and test results, as well as phone calls regarding medical advice. In Japan, the rates of consultations are high because doctors not only prescribe but also dispense medication.

Chapter 11

MEDICAL DOCTORS IN THE FOCUS OF ATTENTION AND OF CONTRADICTORY INTERESTS IN HEALTH CARE

The relationship between doctor and patient is often characterised by contradictory pressures and differences in interests. When problems arise relative to the provision of health care, in many countries the blame for current deficiencies is placed on the medical doctor; in other countries, the problem becomes a political football, with each of the major political parties blaming the other for current shortcomings. The influence of political decision-making is often underestimated, although new laws and legislation often have a significant impact on the daily tasks of the medical practitioner, particularly in terms of administrative paperwork. One of the major shortcomings of new regulations that affect clinical practice is the lack of allowance for changing social and demographic influences as well as economic factors; the elderly inevitably need more care, and an aging population thus implies an increased need for medical services. Difficulties may also arise if the balance between hospital care and private practice is affected: in some systems, large government or privately funded organisations with a professional secretariat are increasingly providing multifaceted outpatient treatment (including advice on diet, lifestyle and psychological problems) and are seen to be competing "unfairly" with long-established but much smaller, independent private practices. As a result, physicians practicing in their own premises experience major anxieties about the future of practices in which they (and sometimes the parents) have invested both their capital and their lives.

In hospitals, too, many medical administrators and other senior medical consultants are experiencing increasing pressures related to their achieving specified administrative and financial goals ranging from minimum waiting times for admission or treatment of surgical conditions to the containment of budgetary shortfalls. They face also the rivalry that develops between competing medical specialties and between doctors working in private practices compared with those employed within a medical institute; these tensions make it difficult to advocate a unified and effective strategy to ameliorate the stressors affecting the various physicians concerned.

A growing number of medical graduates appear to be resolving these dilemmas by moving towards non-clinical and non-curative areas of work. Another personal expression of dissatisfaction with working conditions is emigration. The continuing loss of physicians from developing countries is a major strain on their already tightly-stretched health care budgets. Some developed societies also experience a systematic emigration - for instance, from Canada to larger and more prestigious hospitals in the U.S. Germany also loses a substantial number of its doctors through "emigration". In 2008, 3065 practicing physicians left Germany – the figure was 2439 in the year 2007 – and only 1350 foreign-trained doctors were newly registered in Germany (Kopetsch 2009). Apparently, many experienced physicians and consultants remain dissatisfied with the prospects for personal and professional development in their home country and see little prospect of major and effective reforms. Younger doctors often seem to emigrate because of escalating economic pressures within both private practice and established hospitals, and the ever-growing flood of bureaucracy with which the current generation of physicians must contend. They seek openings abroad which appear to offer them prospects for improved patient care and better niches for reaching their own needs and expectations (Rohbold, 2009).

Chapter 12

CONCLUSIONS

A good physician will not only demonstrate a solid grounding in evidence-based medicine, but will also take due account of anthropologic and cultural factors influencing the needs of individual patients. Often, such an orientation will be reflected in an emphasis on preventive medicine, empathy, a listening ear and the use of simple psychology rather than a reliance on detailed background knowledge of surgery or pharmacology. Patients often have well developed views on factors that are crucial to their satisfaction **as "consumers," although the** meeting of such expectations does not always equate closely with the delivery of quality medical care. From the viewpoint of the physician, the quality of practice is likely to be enhanced by a consideration of personal motivations and factors enhancing job satisfaction; it is also important to assess and where possible to minimize job stressors, seeking to match individual physicians to the various demands of a particular specialty and encouraging appropriate social interaction with members of the growing multidisciplinary medical team. The growing cost of health care in most nations calls for critical choices on optimal methods of treatment and reimbursement, with difficult decisions on economically sustainable levels of care. These various issues have important implications for the selection and training of medical students and the nurture of the physicians after their qualification. Several extended quotations summarize some of the major lessons to be drawn from this review:

"My first impulse on meeting someone new is to listen, with as few interruptions as possible... in the era of managed care, with people typically seen .... every fifteen minutes, there is little incentive for uninterrupted listening... It was surprising to me to learn... what a powerful instrument of change listening is.... people in general are starved for the experience of being heard. Most of our entertainment requires only... listening to others. .. Each of our stories deserves to be told, and yet to whom can we tell them?" (p. 128-129, Livingston, 2006).

Yalom's book for a new generation of therapists offers indications of the qualities important in a good doctor. They include being "fellow travellers", engaging the patient, being supportive and displaying empathy, letting the patient matter to you, acknowledging your errors, using the here and now, self-disclosure, transparency and discretion, talking gently and effectively about life-meaning and death, encouraging self-monitoring, willingness to touch the patient, taking an adequate history, interviewing significant others, and being aware of occupational hazards (Yalom, 2002). Perhaps these are the markers that Osler implied when he distinguished good from great physicians.

REFERENCES

A'Brook, M. (1990). The doctor's health. Psychosis and depression. *Practitioner, 234* (1496), 992–993.

Allibone, A., Oakes, D., & Shannon, H.S. (1981). The health and health care of doctors. *Journal of the Royal College of General Practitioners, 31*, 728-734.

Antoniou, AS., Cooper, C.L., & Davidson, M.J. (2008). A qualitative study investigating gender differences in primary work stressors and levels of job satisfaction in Greek junior doctors. *The Qualitative Report Volume, 13* (3), 456-473.

Ashcroft, R.E. (2002). Searching for the good doctor. *British Medical Journal, 325*, 719.

Ashworth, M., Medina, J., Morgan, M. (2008). Effect of social deprivation on blood pressure monitoring and control in England: a survey of data from the quality and outcomes framework. *British Medical Journal, 337*, 1235-1238.

Aswani, V. (2001) Empathy development in physicians. *Medscape Medical Students.*

Australian Medical Association Ltd. (2006). Health and Well-being of medical students and practitioners.

Baker, R. (2006). Developing standards, criteria, and thresholds to assess fitness to practise. *British Medical Journal, 332*, 230.

Banjo, J. (2007). Medical Errors and Medical Narcissism ... 2 years later. Health Care Ethics Consortium of Georgia. Emory University.

Belfer, B. (1989). Stress and the medical practitioner. *Stress Health , 5* (2), 109-113.

Bissel, L., & Jones, R.W. (1976). The alcoholic practitioner: A survey. *American Journal of Psychiatry, 133*, 1142.

Björnberg, A., & Uhlir, M. (2008). *Euro Health Consumer Index 2008*. Health Consumer Powerhouse AB.

British Medical Journal Editor (2008). Healthy doctors - Healthy practice. *British Medical Journal, 337,* 1121-1122.

Bogue, R.J., Gaueneri, J.G., Reed, M., Bradley, K., & Hughes, J. (2006). Secrets of physician satisfaction: Study identifies pressure points and reveals life practices of highly satisfied doctors. *The Physician Executive, Nov/Dec,* 30-33.

Brooke, D., Edwards, S.G., & Taylor, C. (1991). Addiction as an occupational hazard. *British Journal of Addiction, 86,* 1011-1016.

Buddeberg-Fischer, B., Stamm, M., Buddeberg, C., & Klaghofer, R. (2008). The new generation of family physicians – career motivation, life goals and work-life balance. *Swiss Medical Weekly, 138,* 21-22, 305-312.

Caplan, R.P. (1994). Stress, anxiety and depression in hospital consultants, general practitioners, and senior health service managers. *British Medical Journal, 309,* 1261-1263.

Cartwright, L.K. (1987). Occupational stress in women physicians. In Payne, R.L., & Firth-Cozens, J., (Eds.), Stress in the Health professionals, 71-87. Chichester, U.K.: Wiley.

Chambers, R., Wall, D., & Campbell, I. (1996). Stresses, coping mechanisms and job satisfaction in general practitioner registrars. *British Journal of General Practice, 46,* 343-348.

Charon, R. (2001). Narrative medicine. A model of empathy, reflection, profession and trust. *Journal of the American Medical Association, 286,* 1897-1902.

Chen, P.W. (2008, Oct. 23). Stories in the service of making a better doctor. *New York Times.*

Cleary, P.D., Edgman-Levitan, S., Roberts, M., Moloney, T.W., McMullen, W., Walker, J.D., et al. (1991). Data watch. Patients evaluate their hospital care: A National Survey. *Health Affairs, Winter,* 255-267.

Clever, S., Jin, L., Levinson, W., & Meltzer, D.O. (2008). Does doctor-patient communication affect patient satisfaction with hospital care? *Health Service Research, 43* (5), 1505-1519.

Clode, D. (2004). *The conspiracy of silence: Emotional health among medical practitioners.* Melbourne: Royal Australian College of General Practitioners.

Compton Interactive Encyclopaedia (1995). *Women's History in America.* Retrieved from the Women International Centre Web Site: http://www.wic.org/misc/history.htm

Constanti, A., Solano, L., Di Napoli, R., Bosco, A. (1997). Relationship between hardiness and risk of burnout in a sample of 92 nurses working in oncology and AIDS wards. *Psychotherapy & Psychosomatics*, 78-82.

Cooper, C.L., Rout, U., & Faragher, B., (1989). Mental Health, job satisfaction, and job stress among general practitioners. *British Medical Journal, 298*, 366-370.

Cooper, J.B., Newbauer, R.S., Long, C.D., & McPeek, B. (2002). Preventable aesthesia mishaps: A study of human factors. *Quality and Safety in Health Care, 11*, 277-282.

Cruess, S., Cruess, R., Steinert, Y. (2008). Role modelling - Making the most of powerful teaching strategy. *British Medical Journal, 336*, 718-721.

Cumming, A. (2002) Good communication skills can mask deficiencies. *British Medical Journal 325*, 676.

Deveugele, M., Derese, A., van den Brick-Muinen, A., Benzing, J., & De Maeseneer, J. (2002). Consultation length in general practise: Cross sectional study in six European countries. *British Medical Journal, 325*, 472.

Doc Martin. (n.d.) retrieved September 14, 2008. From en.wikipedia.org/wiki/Doc_Martin

Easton, G. (2006). Wanted: Spunky TV doctor. *British Medical Journal, 332*, 1457.

Elliott, G.R., & Eisdorfer, C. (1982). *Stress and Human Health*. New York: Springer Publishing Company.

Ennis, M., & Vincent, C.A. (1990). Obstetric accidents: A review of 64 cases. *British Medical Journal, 300* (6763), 1365-1367.

European Commission EU. (2006). *Meaical errors. Special barometer*, (Publication No. 241). Directorate-General Press and Communication.

European Commission (2007). *Health in the European Union. Special Eurobarometer*, (Publication No. 272e.). Directorate-General Press and Commission.

Ferguson, E., James, D., Madeley, L. (2002). Factors associated with success in medical school and in a medical career: systematic review of the literature. *British Medical Journal, 324*, 952-957.

Forum Gesundheitspolitik. (2009). *Der Frauenanteil unter den Ärzten steigt: Ist dadurch die sprechende Medizin im Kommen?*. Retrieved from http://www.forum-gesundheitspolitik.de/artikel/artikel.pl?artikel=0628

Fuchs, E. (2008). Physicians, medical students struggle with mental illness and suicide. *Association of American Medical Colleges*. Retrieved from: http://www.aamc.org/newsroom/reporter/dec08/mentalillness.htm.

Fung, K. (2007). *Why are we at risk?* Department of Psychiatry University of Alberta.

Furnham, A, (1988) *Lay theories. Everyday understanding of problems in the social sciences. (International Series in Experimental Social Psychology).* Oxford: Pergamon,

Furnham, A.F., & Kirkcaldy, B.D. (1997). Age and sex differences in health beliefs and behaviour. *Psychological Reports, 80,* 63-66.

Furnham, A.F. (1988). *Lay Theories. Everyday understanding of problems in the social sciences.* Oxford: Pergamon Press.

General Medical Council (2001). *Good medical practice.* London: General Medical Council.

Goleman, D. (1996). *Emotional Intelligence. Why it can matter more than IQ.* Bloomsbury, London: Bantam Books.

Gorin Rosenbaum, G.S. (2002). What's a good doctor and how do you make one? Some magic is required. *British Medical Journal, 325,* 711.

Griffith, G., Fox-Rusby, J., Buxton, M., *The cost-effectiveness of population level interventions to lower cholesterol and prevent Coronary Heart Disease: extrapolation and modelling results on promoting healthy eating habits from Norway to the UK* Final Phase 2 Report for the project "Health economic analysis of prevention and intervention approaches to reducing incidence of Coronary Heart Disease".

Groopman, J. (2008). *How doctors think.* New York: Houghton Mifflin

Guthrie, E., & Black, D. (1997). Psychiatric disorder, stress and burnout. *Advances in Psychiatric Treatment, 3,* 275-281.

Harris, P.E. (1989). The Nurse Stress Index. *Work and Stress, 3,* 335-346.

Hayward, R. (2006) Balancing certainty and uncertainty in clinical medicine. *Developmental Medicine and Child Neurology, 48,* 74-77.

Herzig, S., Biehl, L., Stelberg, H., Hick, C., Schmeisser, N., Koerfer, A. (2006). When is a doctor a good doctor? An analysis of the contents of statements by representatives of the medical profession. *Deutsche Medizinische Wochenschrift, 131,* 2883-2888.

Hild, C. (2004). Arctic telehealth: north to the future. *International Journal of Circumpolar Health, 2,* 63-70.

Hurwitz, B., Vass, A. (2002). What's a good doctor, and how can you make one? *British Medical Journal, 325,* 667-668.

Kemsley, R. (2008) Architecture and general practice. *British Journal of General Practice, 58,* 517.

Kirkcaldy, B.D., & Siefen, R.G. (1991). Occupational stress among medical health professionals. *Social Psychiatry and Psychiatric Epidemiology, 26,* 238-244.

Kirkcaldy, B. D., & Cooper, C. L., (1992). Cross-cultural differences in occupational stress among British and German Managers. *Work and Stress, 6* (2), 177-190.

Kirkcaldy, B.D., Furnham, A.F., & Lynn, R.A. (1992). National differences in work attitudes between the UK and Germany. *European Work and Organizational Psychologist, 2* (2), 81-102.

Kirkcaldy, B.D., & Pope, M. (1992) A structural analysis of a psycho-oncology unit. *European Work and Organisational Psychologist, 2* (1), 33-51.

Kirkcaldy, B.D., Pope, M., & Siefen, R.G. (1993). Sociogrid analysis of a child and adolescent psychiatric clinic. *Social Psychiatry and Psychiatric Epidemiology, 28,* 296-303.

Kirkcaldy, B.D., Athanasou, J.A., & Trimpop, R. (2000). The idiosyncratic construction of stress: examples from medical work settings. *Stress Medicine, 16,* 315-326.

Kirkcaldy, B.D., & Shephard, R.J. (2001). Predicting mental and physical health among social and medical professions. *European Review of Applied Psychology, 51* (4), 243-253.

Kirkcaldy, B.D., Brown, Furnham, A., & Trimpop, R. (2002). Job stress and dissatisfaction: Comparing male and female medical practitioners and auxiliary personnel. *European Review of Applied Psychology, 52* (1), 51-61.

Kirkcaldy, B.D., Shephard, R.J., & Furnham, A.F. (2002). The influence of Type A and locus of control upon job satisfaction and occupational health. *Personality and Individual Differences, 33,* 1361-1371.

Kirkcaldy, B.D., & Siefen, R.G. (2002). The occupational stress and health outcome profiles of clinical directors in child and adolescent psychiatry. *Stress and health, 18,* 161-172.

Kirkcaldy, B.D., & Siefen, G. (2005). Investment in health care and psychological and physical well-being in European nations. In: M.H. Smyth (Ed.), *Health care issues.* New York: Nova Science Publishers.

Kirkcaldy, B.D., Siefen, R.G., Merbach, M., Rutow, N., Brähler, E., & Wittig, U. (2007). A comparison of general and illness-related locus of control in russians, ethnic german migrants and germans. *Psychology, Health and Medicine, 12* (3), 364-379.

Kirkcaldy, B.D., Trimpop, R.T., & Martin, T., (2009). Characteristics of the job and its impact on psychosocial well-being among the medical professions. (submitted)

Kmietowicz, Z. (2006). Patients' views on access will affect GPs' pay. *British Medical Journal, 333*, 1137.

Kopetsch, T. (2009). Arztzahlentwicklung: Hohe Abwanderung ins Ausland – sehr geringe Arbeitslosigkeit. *Deutsches Ärzteblatt 106* (16) A757 – A760, 2009.

Kuusela, M., Vainiomki, P., Hinkka, S., Rautava, P. (2004). The quality of GP consultation in two different salary systems. *Scandinavian Journal of Primary Health Care, 22*, 168-173.

Leue, C., van Os., J., Neeleman, J., de Graf, R., Vollebergh, W., & Stockbrügger, R.W. (2005). Bidirectional associations between depression/anxiety and bowel diseases in a population based cohort. *Journal of Epidemiology and Community Health, 59*, 434.

Lievens, F., Coelsier, P., De Frayt, F., & De Maeseneer, J. (2002). Medical students' personality characteristics and academic performance: a five-factor model perspective . *Medical Education, 36* (11), 1050-1056.

Lindeman, S., Laara, G., Hakko, H., & Lonnqvist, J. (1996). A systematic review on gender, specific suicide mortality in medical doctors. *British Journal of Psychiatry, 168*, 274-279.

Livingston, G. (2006). *And never stop dancing. Thirty more true things you need to know now*. New York: Marlowe and Co.

Lown, B. (1999). *The lost art of healing. Practising compassion in medicine*. New York: Ballantine Books.

McCranie, E.W., Brandsma, J.M., (1988). Personality antecedents of burnout among middle-aged physicians. *Journal of Behavioural Medicine, 11*, 30-36.

McLellan, A.T., Skipper, G.S., Campbell, M., Dupont, R.L. (2008). Five year outcomes in a cohort study of physicians treated for substance use disorders in the United States. *British Medical Journal, 337*, 1154-1156.

McManus, I.C. (1982). A level grades and medical school admission. *British Medical Journal, 284*, 1654.

Mossialos, A. (1996). *Satisfaction in health care systems*. Brussels: European Union.

Murray, R.M. (1977). Psychiatric illness in male doctors and controls: An analysis of Scottish inpatient data. *British Journal of Psychiatry, 131*, 1-10.

Newton, B. W., Barber, L., Clardy, J., Cleveland, E., & O'Sullivan, P. (2008) Is there hardening of the heart during medical school? *Academic Medicine, 83* (3), 244-249.

Odberg, M.H., Eriksen, T.R., & Petersson, B.H. (1995). The effect of gender on the physician role. Attitudes and expectations of medical students examined

by a questionnaire at the start of their studies. *Ugeskr Laeger, 4*, 157, 36, 4942-6.
Organisation for Economic Co-Operation and Development (2003). OECD Health Indicator, Vol. 1. *Organisation for Economic Cooperation and Development.* Paris : OECD.
Organisation for Economic Co-Operation and Development: Health Data (2008). *Public satisfaction and health care systems.* Paris : OECD.
Organisation for Economic Co-Operation and Development (2008). *Policy Brief. Organisation for Economic Cooperation and Development.* Paris : OECD.
Organisation for Economic Co-Operation and Development (2008). *OECD Health Data.* Paris : OECD.
Paice, E., Heard, S., & Moss, F. (2002). How important are role models in making good doctors? *British Medical Journal, 325,* 707-710.
Peterkin, A. (2009). *Resident health: Risks and challenges.* [PowerPoint slides] Retrieved from: hsl.mcmaster.ca/medicine/unit6/allanpeterkin.ppt
Pillay, R. (2008). Work satisfaction of medical doctors in the South African private health sector. *Journal of Health Organisation and Management, 22* (3), 254-268.
Potiriadis, M., Chondros, P., Gilchrist, C. (2008). How do Australian patients rate their general practitioner? A descriptive study using the General Practice Assessment Questionnaire. *Medical Journal of Australia, 189,* 215-219.
Ray, C., & Baum, M. (1985). *Psychological aspects of early breast cancer.* New York: Springer Verlag.
Registrar General (1978). *Decennial supplement for England and Wales.* London: HMSO.
Richardsen, A.M., & Burke, R.J. (1991). Occupational stress and job satisfaction among middle-aged physicians: Sex differences. *Social Sciences and Medicine, 33,* 1179-1187.
Rinpoche, C.D., & Shlim, D.R. (2006). Medicine and compassion. A tibetan lama's guidance for caregivers. Massachusetts: Wisdome
Robertson, R., Dixon, A., Le Grand, J. (2008). Patient choice in general practice: the implications of patient satisfaction surveys. *Journal of Health Service Research & Policy, 13,* 67-72.
Robold, C. (2009) Offener Brief eines Auswanderers. Sehr geehrte Frau Ministerin, ich gehe als Arzt nach Neuseeland (Dear Minister, I am going to work as a doctor in New Zealand). *Deutsches Ärzteblatt 106* (21), A1073 – A1074, 2009

Rode, A., Shephard, R.J., Vloshinsky, P.E., Kuksis, A. (1995). Plasma fatty acid profiles of Canadian inuit and Siberian ganasan. *Artic Medical Research, 54*, 10-20.

Royal College of General Practitioners. Good medical practice for general practitioners. London: RCGP, 2002.

Royal College of Physicians (2006) Briefly on women in Medicine. Retrieved from:
http://www.rcplondon.ac.uk/college/statements/briefing_womenmed.asp.

Rucinski, T., & Cybulska, E. (1985). Mentally ill doctors. *British Journal of Hospital Medicine, 43*, 90-94.

Rudland, J.R., & Mires, G. (2005). Characteristics of doctors and nurses as perceived by students entering medical school: Implications for shared teaching. *Medical Education, 39* (5), 448-455.

Rø, K.E.I., Gude, T., Tyssen, R., Aasland, O.G. (2008). Counselling for burnout in Norwegian doctors: One year cohort study. *British Medical Journal, 337*, 1146-1149.

Sawicki, P., Bastian, H. (2008). German health care: A bit of Bismarck plus more science. *British Medical Journal, 337*, 1142-1145.

Schattner, P.I., & Colman, G.S. (1998). The stress of metropolitan general practices. *Medical Journal of Australia, 169*, 133-137.

Schwartz, B. (2005). *The paradox of choice. Why more is less*. New York: Harper

Shephard, R.J. (1996). Habitual physical activity and the quality of life. *Quest, 48*, 354-365.

Shephard, R.J., Rode, A. (1996). *The health consequences of 'modernization'*. Cambridge: Cambridge University Press.

Shernhammer, E.S., & Colditz, G.A. (2004). Suicide rates among physicians: A quantitative and gender assessment (meta-analysis). *American Journal of Psychiatry, 161* (12), 2295-2302.

Sinclair, J., Lawson, B., Burge, F. (2008). Which patients receive advice on diet and exercise? Do certain characteristics affect whether they receive such advice. *Canadian Family Physician, 54*, 404-412.

Sokol, D. (2004, June 29). Truth is not always the best medicine. Retrieved from the International Herald Tribune's Web Site: http://www.nytimes.com/2004/06/29/opinion/29iht-edsokol_ed3__0.html.

Sokol, D.K., (2008). Medicine as performance: what can magicians teach doctors? *Journal of Royal Social Medicine 101*, 443-446.

Sutherland, V.J., & Cooper, C.L. (1992). Job stress, satisfaction, and mental health among general practitioners before and after introduction of new contact. *British Medical Journal, 304*, 1545-1548.

Sutherland, V.J. & Cooper, C.L. (1993) Identifying distress among general practitioners: Predictors of psychological ill-health and job dissatisfaction. *Social Science and Medicine, 37*, 575-581

Symons, L., & Persuade, R. (1995). Stress among doctors. *British Medical Journal, 310,* 742.

Taleb, N.N. (2007) *The Black Swan. The impact of the highly improbable.* Penguin, London.

Tavris, C., & Aronson, E. (2007). *Mistakes were made (but not by me). Why we justify foolish beliefs, bad decisions, and hurtful acts.* New York: Harvest Book/Harcourt.

Tetrick, L.E., Quick, J.C., & Quick, J.D. (2005). Prevention perspectives in occupational health psychology. In: A.S.G. Antoniou & C.L. Cooper (Eds.). *Research Companion to Organizational health Psychology,* p. 209-217. Cheltenham, U.K.: Edward Elgar Publishers

UK Department of Health (2003). *Investing in general practice: The new GMS contract.* London, UK: Department of Health.

Van Dam, R.M., Spiegelman, D., Franco, O.H., & Hu, B.H. (2008). Combined impact of lifestyle factors on mortality: Prospective cohort study in US women. *British Medical Journal, 337*, 440.

Vincent, C., & Furnham, A. (1997). *Complementary Medicine. A Research Perspective.* Chichester, England: Wiley.

Wakeford, R. (2006). Criteria, competencies and confidence tricks. *British Medical Journal, 332,* 233.

World Health Organization (2009). *Suicide.* Retrieved from: www.who.inter/mental_health/prevention/suicide

Yalom, I.D. (2002). *The gift of therapy. An open letter to a new generation of therapists and their patients.* New York: Harper-Collins.

Zelnio, D. (2009). *The Changing Face of Medicine.* Retrieved from: www.mommd/changingfacehealthcare.html

CONTRIBUTORS

Bruce Kirkcaldy has academic degrees in psychology from the Universities of Dundee (UK) and Giessen (Germany), as well as postgraduate professional training as a behavioural therapist and clinical psychologist. He is Director of the International Centre for the Study of Occupational and Mental Health, Moderator for post professional training groups in Psychotherapy and Psychological Health, and runs his own psychotherapy practise specialising in the treatment of anxiety and depressive disorders and psychosomatic ailments. He has published some 200 articles including several edited books, with research and writing interests directed towards clinical and health issues and organisational and leisure psychology. Currently he is on the editorial board of several health and management journals as well as occasional reviewer for some 20 medical health and psychology journals. Email contact: brucedavidkirkcaldy@yahoo.de

Roy Shephard has graduate and post-graduate degrees in Medicine from the University of London, and a Doctorate in Physiology. After a brief period in the department of Cardiology at Guy's Hospital (where he was responsible primarily for the cardiac catheterisation of patients with congenital heart disease), he embarked on a research career in cardio-respiratory and exercise physiology. Much of his career was spent at the University of Toronto, serving as a Professor in the Departments of Physiology and Preventive Medicine, and the School of Physical Education and Health. For many years, he was Director of that School and of the Graduate Programme in Exercise Sciences. Email contact is: royjshep@shaw.ca

Rainer G. Siefen served as the Medical Director of the Westfalia Clinic for Child and Adolescent Psychiatry for many years and is currently Head of the Unit for Psychosomatics at the Department of Paediatrics at St. Josef Hospital at the

Ruhr University Bochum. He graduated in medicine and went onto study psychology. He is a specialist in child and adolescent psychiatry and is a psychiatrist and neurologist as well as a practising psychotherapist. His major research interests include migration and health, drug and alcohol abuse among children and adolescence, eating disorders, and the relationships between parents and their children. Germany. Email: r.siefen@klinikum-bochum.de

INDEX

A

academic performance, 68
accessibility, 20, 38
accidents, 51, 65
achievement, 32, 44, 49
acid, 70
acute, 4, 15
adaptation, 3
administration, 29, 31, 32, 34
administrative, 30, 31, 32, 49, 51, 59, 60
administrators, 19, 31, 33, 60
adolescence, 74
adult, 14, 37
adult population, 14
adults, 38
age, 55, 57
agents, 4, 15, 37
aging, 33, 59
aging population, 33, 59
agreeableness, 32
AIDS, 47, 65
air, 30, 55
Alberta, 66
alcohol, 48, 51, 74
alcohol abuse, 74
alcohol dependence, 51
alcohol use, 48
altruism, 45
ambiguity, 49
antecedents, 3, 68
antidepressants, 15
anxiety, 8, 13, 15, 19, 45, 51, 54, 64, 68, 73
anxiety disorder, 51
appetite, 4
Arctic, 66
arthritis, 8
assault, 48, 54
assertiveness, 49
assessment, 1, 33, 70
asthma, 8
attacks, 5
attitudes, 9, 17, 18, 25, 43, 46, 54, 67
aura, 22, 54
Australia, 9, 69, 70
Austria, 8, 9, 14, 20, 57
authority, 5, 29
autonomy, 18, 26, 28, 30
availability, 30, 57
awareness, 5, 52

B

Bayesian analysis, 42
behavioral disorders, 16
behaviours, 43
Belgium, 7, 9, 14, 15, 20, 37
beliefs, 7, 17, 18, 19, 57, 66, 71
benchmarking, 2
benefits, 4, 18, 24, 33

bias, 4, 51
bipolar, 51
bipolar disorder, 51
birth, 35, 37
births, 37
blame, 59
blaming, 59
blood, 1, 8, 34, 55, 63
blood pressure, 34, 55, 63
body mass index, 34
borderline, 51
bowel, 68
Brazil, 37
breast cancer, 69
breathing, 16
bronchitis, 8
Brussels, 68
Bulgaria, 8, 20
bureaucracy, 60
Burkina Faso, 37
burn, 47
burnout, 26, 47, 65, 66, 68, 70

C

Canada, 35, 37, 38, 39, 55, 60
cancer, 4, 8
candidates, 26, 41, 42
cardiologist, 23
cardiovascular disease, 4
caregivers, 47, 69
causality, 37
Central America, 37
Central Europe, 8
childbirth, 54
children, 19, 21, 38, 74
cholesterol, 66
chronic disease, 4, 16
chronic diseases, 4
cigarette smoking, 5
cirrhosis, 51
classroom, 42
clinics, 43, 49, 55
Co, 64, 68, 69
cohort, 68, 70, 71

colleges, 44
communication, 18, 21, 31, 32, 35, 44, 49, 54, 64, 65
communication skills, 18, 21, 44, 65
communities, 4
community, 1, 42
compassion, 23, 43, 44, 45, 68, 69
compatibility, 23
competence, 19, 23, 28, 32, 42, 45, 52
competency, 29
competition, 26, 30
competitiveness, 9
complexity, 34
compliance, 17, 18, 54
components, 17
comprehension, 45
computerization, 3
conditioning, 30
confidence, 19, 53, 54, 71
confinement, 17
confrontation, 57
congenital heart disease, 73
conscientiousness, 32
consensus, 18
conspiracy, 64
constraints, 31, 52
construction, 67
consultants, 30, 50, 60, 64
consulting, 57
consumers, 28, 61
consumption, 19
control, 5, 38, 49, 51, 63, 67
control group, 51
coping strategies, 31
coronary heart disease, 4
correlation, 35, 37
correlations, 35, 42
cost-effective, 66
costs, 18, 31, 33, 40, 57
creativity, 23
credit, 52
criticism, 18
Croatia, 20
crops, 3
cross-cultural differences, 2

Cuba, 37, 38, 39
cues, 18, 31
cultivation, 3
cultural beliefs, 57
cultural differences, 42, 67
cultural factors, 61
culture, 7, 20, 21, 54
curing, 16
currency, 37
curriculum, 43, 45
Czech Republic, 9, 57

distress, 71
distribution, 34, 37
diversity, 34
doctor-patient, 43, 45, 64
doctors, 4, 9, 18, 19, 21, 26, 29, 30, 31, 32, 33, 37, 41, 43, 44, 45, 49, 50, 51, 52, 53, 54, 55, 57, 60, 63, 64, 66, 68, 69, 70, 71
dosage, 9, 10, 11, 54
drug abuse, 51
drugs, 4, 9, 11, 18, 37, 55
duration, 20, 34, 54

D

danger, 21, 51, 55
death, 30, 47, 53, 62
death rate, 30
deaths, 4
decision-making process, 30, 31
decisions, 18, 38, 40, 48, 53, 61, 71
deficit, 15
delivery, 55, 61
denial, 53
Denmark, 7, 8, 9, 20, 37, 54
density, 34, 57
dentists, 41
depressed, 27
depression, 8, 13, 15, 37, 50, 51, 63, 64, 68
depressive disorder, 15, 73
deprivation, 63
detection, 18
developing countries, 60
diabetes, 8
diet, 3, 4, 21, 31, 34, 43, 59, 70
diets, 3
differential rates, 57
diffusion, 19
disability, 37
disappointment, 52
discipline, 32
disclosure, 24, 54, 62
discomfort, 18, 21
diseases, 4, 68
disorder, 15, 66
dissatisfaction, 20, 30, 60, 67

E

early retirement, 28
earnings, 51
eating, 66, 74
eating disorders, 74
Education, 40, 68, 70, 73
educators, 45
e-health, 20
elderly, 59
emigration, 60
emotional distress, 51
emotional exhaustion, 48
Emotional Intelligence, 66
emotional state, 13
emotions, 13
empathy, 19, 23, 32, 43, 44, 45, 47, 52, 61, 62, 64
emphysema, 8
employment, 9, 41, 44
empowerment, 31
endurance, 44
engagement, 31
England, 63, 69, 71
entertainment, 62
enthusiasm, 43
environment, 3, 21, 30, 49
Estonia, 7, 20
ethanol, 51
ethics, 33
Euro, 64
European Commission, 7, 65
European Union (EU), 8, 14, 20, 53, 65, 68

78   Index

Europeans, 14, 15
evolution, 4
examinations, 24, 32, 42, 45
excuse, 54
exercise, 3, 70, 73
expenditures, 2, 16, 33, 35, 37, 38, 39, 40, 55
expertise, 14
exposure, 44
extrapolation, 66
extraversion, 32

F

failure, 55
family, vii, 2, 9, 13, 15, 18, 26, 29, 30, 44, 45, 49, 52, 64
family medicine, 9, 45
family physician, 2, 13, 29, 64
fatigue, 47
fatty acid, 4, 70
fatty acids, 4
fear, 30, 48, 54
fears, 17, 54
fee, 30, 38, 39, 44
feelings, 47
fees, 57
females, 51
film, 1
Finland, 8, 15, 20, 37, 54
fishing, 1
fitness, 63
five-factor model, 68
flood, 60
food, 3, 4
food intake, 4
food products, 3
football, 59
forceps, 54
Fox, 34, 66
fractures, 16
France, 9, 14, 15, 20, 37, 41, 57
freedom, 30, 34
Freud, 44

G

GDP, 35, 37, 39
gender, 9, 15, 26, 63, 68, 70
gender differences, 9, 15, 26, 63
general practitioner, 1, 9, 14, 15, 29, 30, 48, 50, 54, 57, 64, 65, 69, 70, 71
general practitioners, 9, 29, 30, 48, 50, 54, 64, 65, 70, 71
generation, 3, 44, 60, 62, 64, 71
Georgia, 63
Germany, 8, 9, 20, 34, 35, 37, 41, 55, 57, 60, 67, 73, 74
gift, 71
GNP, 35
goals, 2, 41, 60, 64
government, iv, 59
GPs, 19, 29, 50, 68
grades, 32, 42, 68
gravitation, 50
Great Britain, 15
Greece, 8, 15, 16, 20, 37, 56, 57
grief, 16
grounding, 61
groups, 2, 7, 30, 33, 44, 49, 51, 73
growth, 30
guidance, 69
guidelines, 24, 38

H

habitat, 4
Haiti, 37, 39
half-life, 52
happiness, 30, 35, 37
hazards, 62
healing, 16, 22, 68
health care, 5, 17, 18, 19, 20, 21, 31, 33, 34, 35, 38, 49, 55, 59, 60, 61, 63, 67, 68, 69, 70
health care professionals, 5, 49
health care system, 20, 31, 35, 38, 55, 68, 69
health expenditure, 35
health insurance, 31, 34
health services, 35

heart, 4, 16, 43, 45, 54, 66, 68, 73
heart attack, 5
heart disease, 5
helplessness, 47
high blood pressure, 8
high scores, 49
homogenisation, 38
honesty, 23, 24
hopelessness, 47
hospital, 21, 29, 30, 31, 32, 33, 34, 35, 42, 43, 45, 49, 53, 55, 59, 64
hospital beds, 34, 35
hospital care, 34, 59, 64
hospitals, 30, 33, 38, 44, 60
host, 16, 21
human, 3, 38, 47, 53, 65
humanism, 45
humanity, 23
humans, 3
humiliation, 54
Hungarians, 8
Hungary, 7, 9, 16, 20, 54, 57
hunting, 3
hypertension, 4, 8

I

id, 21, 29, 37
identification, 47
illusion, 13
immigrants, 18
impairments, 8
implementation, 43
in situ, 47
inattention, 21
incentive, 61
incentives, 21, 30, 33
incidence, 16, 48, 66
income, 9, 25, 30, 51
incomes, 54
independence, 26
indices, 38
infant mortality, 20, 34, 35, 37, 38, 39
infant mortality rate, 20
infants, 34

infection, 27
infectious diseases, 4
injury, iv
insight, 45
insomnia, 15
instruction, 21, 43, 52
insurance, 31, 33, 35
insurance companies, 31, 34
integrity, 43
intellectual skills, 18
interaction, 30, 61
interactions, 30, 40, 51
internists, 54
interpersonal skills, 32
intervention, 33, 66
intrinsic motivation, 42
IQ, 66
Ireland, 8, 15, 20, 56
irrationality, 53
Israel, 37, 41
Italy, 8, 14, 15, 16, 20, 37, 56

Japan, 16, 37, 57
job dissatisfaction, 30, 48, 71
job satisfaction, 29, 30, 31, 42, 49, 61, 63, 64, 65, 67, 69
judge, 1, 19
judgment, 24, 53
jurisdictions, 19
justice, 23

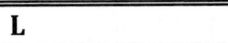

King, 17
Korea, 16, 37, 56

L

lack of opportunities, 49
lactose, 4
land, 13
language, 7, 12

large-scale, 49
Latvia, 7, 20
laws, 59
lawsuits, 25
lawyers, 38
learning, 29, 42, 43, 44, 52
learning process, 43
legislation, 59
leisure, 31, 73
liberal, 44
life expectancy, 34, 35, 37, 38
life span, 34, 57
lifestyle, 2, 3, 4, 5, 33, 34, 47, 52, 59, 71
likelihood, 8, 15, 18
limitations, 23, 25, 31
listening, 1, 31, 43, 44, 52, 61
Lithuania, 7
litigation, 51, 54
locus, 5, 49, 67
London, 41, 66, 69, 70, 71, 73
loneliness, 48
long work, 44
longevity, 39
longitudinal study, 4, 32
Luxemburg, 7, 9, 15, 20, 57

M

Macedonia, 20
maintenance, 40, 55
Maintenance, 47, 55
major decisions, 53
major depression, 51
males, 51
malpractice, 25, 27, 54
Malta, 8
management, 2, 31, 38, 46, 49, 54, 73
market, 19
marriage, 21
marriages, 45
mask, 22, 35, 65
Massachusetts, 69
maternal, 37, 38, 39
measures, 22, 23, 46, 49
media, 30, 45, 48

medical care, 2, 18, 19, 29, 31, 34, 40, 43, 57, 61, 65
medical school, 4, 5, 26, 41, 42, 43, 45, 65, 68, 70
medical services, 20, 33, 40, 59
medical student, 26, 32, 40, 41, 42, 43, 45, 52, 61, 63, 65, 68
Medicare, 28
medication, 15, 21, 30, 34, 37, 51, 54, 57
medications, 9, 37
medicine, 1, 3, 4, 15, 16, 18, 21, 23, 26, 31, 32, 41, 42, 44, 45, 47, 52, 53, 55, 61, 64, 66, 68, 69, 70, 74
Mediterranean, 8
Mediterranean countries, 8
men, 14, 26, 29, 37, 41
mental disorder, 9, 14, 37
mental health, 8, 14, 15, 51, 70
mental illness, 16, 65
mentorship, 52
messages, 5
meta-analysis, 70
metabolizing, 4
methamphetamine, 15
Mexico, 16, 37, 57
middle-aged, 4, 68, 69
migraine, 8
migrants, 67
migration, 74
milk, 4
misleading, 53
mobility, 8
models, 7, 43, 69
modernization, 70
money, 26, 57
morale, 49
morbidity, 8
mortality, 20, 34, 35, 37, 38, 39, 68, 71
motivation, 17, 26, 42, 64
multidisciplinary, 18, 29, 32, 61
myocardial infarction, 20

N

narcissism, 54

narcolepsy, 15
nation, 34, 35
national expenditure, 55
national product, 34
natural food, 3
negative attitudes, 47
neglect, 50
Netherlands, 7, 8, 9, 14, 15, 20, 37, 57
network, 29, 49, 52
neurologist, 74
New York, 64, 65, 66, 67, 68, 69, 70, 71
New York Times, 64
New Zealand, 57, 69
Newton, 45, 68
NHS, 57
Nicaragua, 37
Nobel Prize, 44
non-smokers, 5
normal, 21, 25
norms, 55
North America, 25, 37, 42, 43
Norway, 9, 37, 56, 66
nurse, 13, 35
nurses, 13, 21, 32, 33, 51, 65, 70
nursing, 32
nutrition, 52

O

obese, 55
obesity, 4
obligation, 54
occupational health, 67, 71
OECD, 9, 10, 11, 16, 20, 34, 35, 36, 56, 57, 69
oil, 37
oncology, 47, 65, 67
openness, 43
oppression, 21
optimism, 23
organic disease, 2, 13
orientation, 44, 61
orthodox, 18
osteoporosis, 8
outpatient, 43, 59

overload, 51
overweight, 4
ownership, 25

P

pain, 21, 48
palliative care, 57
paradox, 70
parameter, 21
parents, 26, 32, 59, 74
Paris, 10, 11, 36, 69
passive, 16
patient care, 44, 60
patient rights, 20
patients, vii, 1, 2, 3, 4, 9, 12, 13, 15, 18, 19, 20, 21, 24, 26, 28, 29, 30, 34, 39, 42, 43, 45, 48, 51, 52, 53, 54, 55, 57, 61, 69, 70, 71, 73
peer, 24, 30, 52
peers, 2, 9, 49, 52
peptic ulcer, 8
per capita, 34, 37, 39
per capita expenditure, 34
perception, 19, 29, 53
perceptions, 8, 17, 29, 30, 32
performance indicator, 20
personal control, 5
personal life, 2, 43
personal problems, 50
personal qualities, 2
personal relations, 2
personal relationship, 2
personal responsibility, 19
personality, 17, 42, 44, 50, 51, 53, 68
personality characteristics, 44, 68
personality disorder, 51
personality type, 42, 50
pharmaceutical, 9, 37
pharmaceuticals, 20
pharmacology, 61
philosophy, 44
phone, 23, 57
physical activity, 3, 4, 5, 34, 43, 49, 70
physical exercise, 5

physical health, 5, 48, 67
physical well-being, 67
physicians, 1, 9, 12, 13, 18, 19, 24, 25, 26, 27, 29, 31, 32, 34, 36, 37, 41, 43, 44, 45, 48, 49, 51, 52, 54, 57, 59, 60, 61, 62, 63, 64, 65, 68, 69, 70
physiology, 73
placebo, 22
placebos, 7
plaques, 5
play, 13, 18, 43, 57
poisoning, 51
policy makers, 2, 31
political parties, 59
politicians, 33
poor, 4, 21, 30, 34, 37, 39
population, 2, 4, 9, 14, 33, 34, 35, 36, 38, 48, 51, 57, 59, 66, 68
population group, 33
population size, 9
Portugal, 8, 9, 15, 20, 57
positive attitudes, 5
positive correlation, 14
positive relation, 30
positive relationship, 30
posttraumatic stress, 16
power, 31
predictors, 17, 30, 48
preference, 25
pressure, 8, 16, 31, 34, 63, 64
prestige, 26, 30
prevention, 4, 66, 71
preventive medicine, 3, 4, 55, 61
primary care, 20, 38, 54
private, 13, 38, 39, 57, 59, 60, 69
private practice, 59, 60
professional development, 60
professionalism, 45
professions, 2, 14, 26, 29, 41, 44, 47, 49, 67
prognosis, 7, 12
property, iv
psychiatric disorders, 48
psychiatric illness, 51
psychiatrist, 74
psychiatrists, 15

psychological health, 14, 35, 37, 48, 49
psychological problems, 2, 13, 16, 59
psychological well-being, 5
psychologist, 15, 73
psychology, 13, 14, 43, 61, 71, 73, 74
psychotherapy, 2, 16, 73

Q

quality of life, 23, 34, 70
questioning, 38, 50
questionnaire, 20, 32, 69
questionnaires, 51

R

racism, 21
random, 31
range, 20, 34
ratings, 8, 20, 21, 22, 24, 31
rationality, 26
reading, 45, 52
reality, 24
recession, 33
recognition, 9, 26, 44, 49
reconcile, 9, 44
recovery, 12, 13
recreation, 44
reflection, 64
reforms, 60
regular, 34, 44, 52
regulations, 28, 31, 59
reimbursement, 33, 40, 55, 61
relationship, 1, 2, 13, 17, 18, 21, 37, 38, 43, 45, 49, 52, 53, 55, 59
relationships, 18, 26, 30, 31, 43, 49, 74
relaxation, 49
repair, 21
resolution, 30, 37
resources, 30, 49
respiratory, 73
restructuring, 49
rewards, 34
risk, 4, 34, 44, 46, 47, 48, 51, 65, 66

Index

risk factors, 4, 34
risks, 5, 27, 54
role conflict, 31, 32
Romania, 8, 20

S

salary, 26, 68
sales, 9
sample, 48, 65
satisfaction, 19, 20, 21, 29, 30, 31, 42, 49, 50, 61, 63, 64, 65, 67, 69, 70
school, 4, 5, 26, 41, 42, 43, 45, 65, 68, 70
scores, 8, 20, 21, 35, 45, 49, 50, 51
secretariat, 59
security, 49
sedentary, 5
self-control, 5
self-discipline, 32
self-employment, 44
self-monitoring, 62
sensitivity, 21, 43, 44
services, iv, 19, 20, 33, 35, 55, 57
settlements, 35
severity, 18
sex, 20, 49, 55, 66
sex differences, 66
sexism, 21
sexual activity, 30
shaping, 18
sharing, 32
shoulders, 19
shy, 1
signals, 21
signs, 4
skills, 2, 4, 18, 21, 22, 29, 31, 32, 42, 43, 44, 45, 46, 52, 65
sleep, 15, 30
Slovakia, 8, 20
Slovenia, 54
smokers, 5, 34
smoking, 4, 5
snoring, 16
social class, 51
social context, 33, 39

social fabric, 21
social life, 29
social sciences, 66
social skills, 43, 44
social support, 44, 49
social support network, 49
social work, 26, 51
social workers, 51
sociologists, 17
soft palate, 16
South Africa, 30, 69
Spain, 8, 14, 15, 16, 37
speed, 4
stages, 4
standards, 63
statistics, 34, 38, 51
stereotypes, 32
strain, 60
strategies, 31
stress, 16, 26, 29, 31, 43, 45, 47, 48, 49, 50, 52, 64, 65, 66, 67, 69, 70
stress factors, 52
stressors, 2, 30, 41, 44, 48, 51, 60, 61, 63
strikes, 44
stroke, 8
students, 25, 26, 32, 40, 41, 42, 43, 44, 45, 52, 61, 63, 65, 68, 70
subjective experience, 50
substance abuse, 13, 42
substance use, 68
suburbs, 35
suffering, 47, 48
suicide, 16, 48, 51, 65, 68, 71
suicide rate, 51
supervision, 54
surgery, 15, 18, 30, 54, 55, 61
surgical intervention, 57
susceptibility, 4, 18
Sweden, 7, 9, 20, 37, 57
Switzerland, 9, 20, 35, 37, 56
sympathy, 23, 30
symptom, 18, 42
symptoms, 4, 5, 16, 18, 19

T

tactics, 5
talent, 44
teachers, 51
teaching, 30, 42, 43, 45, 65, 70
technological progress, 52
telehealth, 66
terminally ill, 29
therapeutic relationship, 17
therapists, 62, 71
therapy, 17, 71
thinking, 38, 45, 54, 55
threats, 27, 51
thresholds, 63
time constraints, 52
time pressure, 27
tolerance, 24, 43
trade, 52
tradition, 1
training, 7, 13, 21, 26, 40, 42, 44, 45, 49, 61, 73
traits, 42
transparency, 62
travel, 31
triggers, 31
trust, 1, 19, 64
tundra, 35
Turkey, 37, 57

U

uncertainty, 24, 53, 66
uniform, 34
United Kingdom, 9, 42, 57
United States, 35, 68
universe, 13
university students, 25
urban areas, 20

V

vacation, 26
vaccination, 20
validation, 42
values, 8, 17, 43
variables, 17, 49
village, 1
violence, 21
vulnerability, 13, 15

W

waiting times, 20, 54, 60
Wales, 69
war, 42, 45, 65
well-being, 5, 13, 29, 67
WHO, 16, 37
women, 4, 8, 9, 19, 26, 29, 37, 41, 44, 64, 70, 71
work environment, 29, 31
work ethic, 26
workers, 14, 26, 32
working conditions, 26, 60
working hours, 29, 44
workload, 27, 30, 42, 49
workplace, 49
work-related stress, 25, 47, 49, 50
World Health Organization, 71
writing, vii, 44, 45, 73